About the NCCN Guidelines for Patients®

National Comprehensive Cancer Network®

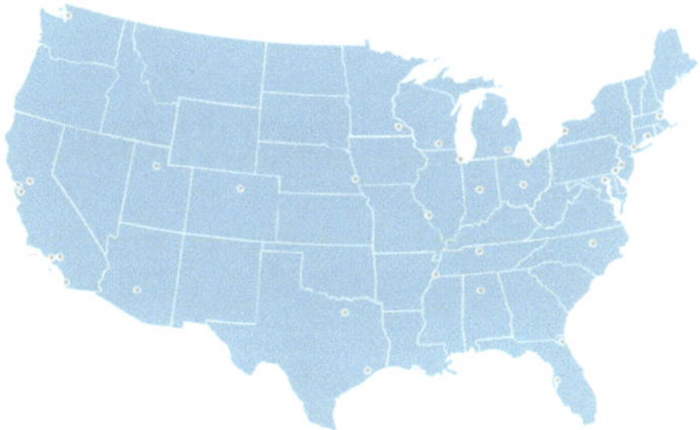

Did you know that top cancer centers across the United States work together to improve cancer care? This alliance of leading cancer centers is called the National Comprehensive Cancer Network® (NCCN®).

Cancer care is always changing. NCCN develops evidence-based cancer care recommendations used by health care providers worldwide. These frequently updated recommendations are the NCCN Clinical Practice Guidelines in Oncology (NCCN Guidelines®). The NCCN Guidelines for Patients plainly explain these expert recommendations for people with cancer and caregivers.

These NCCN Guidelines for Patients are based on the NCCN Clinical Practice Guidelines in Oncology (NCCN Guidelines®) for Melanoma: Cutaneous, Version 2.2025 – January 28, 2025

Learn how the NCCN Guidelines for Patients are developed
NCCN.org/patient-guidelines-process

View the NCCN Guidelines for Patients free online
NCCN.org/patientguidelines

Find an NCCN Cancer Center near you
NCCN.org/cancercenters

Connect with us

Supporters

NATIONAL COMPREHENSIVE CANCER NETWORK®
NCCN FOUNDATION
Guiding Treatment. Changing Lives.

NCCN Guidelines for Patients are supported by funding from the NCCN Foundation®

NCCN Foundation gratefully acknowledges the following corporate supporter for helping to make available these NCCN Guidelines for Patients: Pfizer Inc.

NCCN independently adapts, updates, and hosts the NCCN Guidelines for Patients. Our corporate supporters do not participate in the development of the NCCN Guidelines for Patients and are not responsible for the content and recommendations contained therein.

To make a gift or learn more, visit online or email

NCCNFoundation.org/donate

PatientGuidelines@NCCN.org

Contents

NCCN Foundation seeks to support the millions of patients and their families affected by a cancer diagnosis by funding and distributing NCCN Guidelines for Patients. NCCN Foundation is also committed to advancing cancer treatment by funding the nation's promising doctors at the center of innovation in cancer research. For more details and the full library of patient and caregiver resources, visit NCCN.org/patients.

National Comprehensive Cancer Network (NCCN) and NCCN Foundation
3025 Chemical Road, Suite 100, Plymouth Meeting, PA 19462 USA

1 About melanoma

Melanoma is a serious form of skin cancer. But it is curable, especially if caught early. This patient guideline provides the latest information on melanoma testing, staging, and treatment to help you make informed decisions with your doctor. First, it's important to know what exactly melanoma is and where it starts.

What is melanoma?

Melanoma is one of the most serious types of skin cancer because it spreads beyond the skin more often than many other skin cancers. However, if discovered early, it is curable with the right treatment. More than 3 in 4 are found early — before they have spread — and when they're easier to treat.

Melanoma occurs when something goes wrong in your melanocytes. Melanocytes are skin cells that make melanin, a pigment that gives your skin its color. When skin cells are damaged, new cells may grow out of control and can form a mass of cancerous cells.

Diagnosing and treating melanoma early can lead to better results. It's also encouraging that more effective treatments have become available in the past decade for melanoma that has spread (metastasized).

Important note: While melanoma often occurs in people over 50 years of age, it can

Melanoma skin cancer

Melanoma usually has an irregular shape and different colors. It can show up as a change to an existing mole but also can appear as a new spot on the skin. See Chapter 9 to learn about the ABCDE rule.

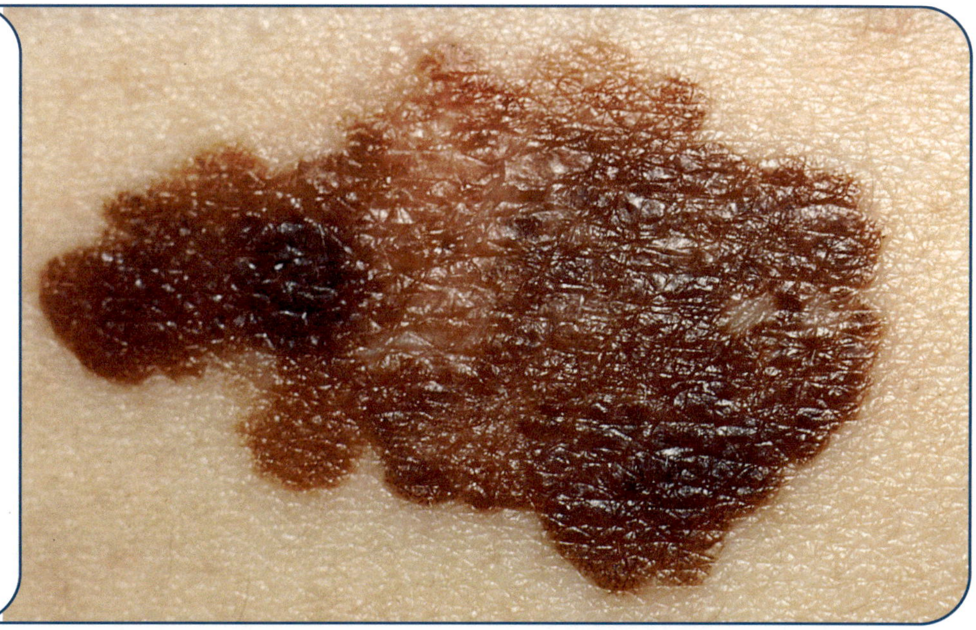

occur in people of younger age — even in children.

Skin basics

Your skin is the largest organ of your body. It covers about 20 square feet — about the size of a dining table top. Skin protects you from invaders (such as bacteria, fungi, and viruses), helps control body temperature, and allows the sensations of touch, heat, and cold.

Skin has 3 layers:

- **Epidermis –** The outermost layer of skin provides a waterproof barrier and creates skin color.
- **Dermis –** This layer contains connective tissue, blood and lymphatic vessels, hair follicles, and sweat glands.
- **Hypodermis –** This deep skin tissue is made of subcutaneous fat, connective tissue, and blood and lymphatic vessels.

Melanin

Melanin is the pigment (chemical) in skin that gives it color. In addition, melanin also protects skin from harmful ultraviolet (UV) rays from the sun. Melanin is produced in cells called melanocytes. Melanocytes are mainly located in the skin at the base of the epidermis. They also determine the color in both your eyes and hair. Melanocytes are found in other areas of the body, but the focus of this book is cancer of sun-exposed and non sun-exposed skin melanocytes, called melanoma.

Causes

It's unclear how damage to cells leads to melanoma. But your genes, your health, and environmental risk factors can all contribute.

Melanoma in the skin

Melanocytes are the cells located in the lower epidermis that when damaged, can become melanoma.

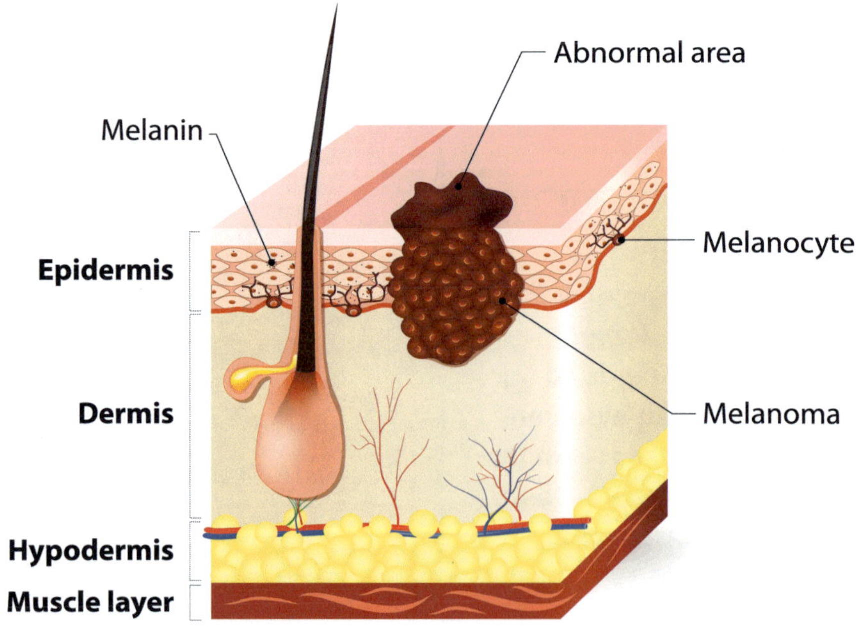

The clearest link is between exposure to UV radiation from the sun or tanning devices. Exposure to UV radiation causes changes to the DNA (genetic material) of pigment cells and increases the risk of melanoma, especially in people with lighter skin tones. It is important to know that UV radiation does not cause all melanomas. Some melanomas can occur in areas of your body that are not exposed to sunlight.

Signs of melanoma

Melanoma lesions (also called tumors) can be found anywhere on your body. Most often, they are found in areas of high-intensity sun exposure such as the trunk, legs, arms, and head. They may appear on normal skin or as a mole that is new or has changed.

Sometimes, melanoma can be found in areas that get little or no sun exposure. These areas can include the soles of your feet, palms of your hands, and underneath your fingernails or toenails (called acral melanomas).

People with darker skin are more likely to develop melanoma in areas that are less exposed to the sun. Melanoma can also occur on internal mucosal surfaces such as in the mouth, inside the nose, on the tongue, or in the intestines (mucosal melanoma); in the genital areas; and in the eyes (ocular or uveal melanoma).

Although rare, melanoma can also show as a bump or a nodule that lacks dark pigment (usually pink or light brown in color), called amelanotic melanoma.

When you or your health care provider examine your skin, attention should be paid to the following:

- A mole that has changed in any way: size, shape, or color
- A new spot on the skin that persists, becomes raised, or bleeds easily
- Ugly duckling sign: a spot that looks different from other spots on your skin

To learn more about spotting melanoma on your own and to learn about the ABCDE rule for moles, see *Chapter 9: Follow-up care*.

Risk factors

The exact cause of melanoma is unknown. But there are many risk factors that make it more likely for you to develop melanoma. A risk factor increases the chance of developing cancer — it doesn't mean you will have melanoma. Some risk factors are associated with activities that people do, like spending time in the sun or tanning devices. Other risk factors are genetic, meaning they are passed down through genes (from parent to child). For more information on genetic risk factors, read *Chapter 9: Follow-up care.*

Here are some of the most common risk factors that make it more likely for a person to develop melanoma:

- **Lighter skin, hair, and eyes** — if you have less melanin (pigment) in your skin, it means less protection from UV radiation. People with light hair and blue/green eyes tend to have less melanin in their skin.

- **A tendency to sunburn** — if you sunburn easily or have a history of chronic sunburns, especially if you develop redness and blistering
- **Many moles** — if you have a high number of moles (more than 50) on your body or they're large and have unusual shapes
- **UV light exposure** — if you spent extended time exposed to UV light (radiation that comes from the sun or tanning devices)
- **Previous skin cancers** — if you have had conditions such as actinic keratosis, or other skin cancers (such as basal cell or squamous cell skin cancers)
- **Childhood cancers** — if you had cancer as a child, this could increase your risk of developing melanoma as you get older
- **Weakened or suppressed immune systems** — if you have a weakened immune system from organ transplants or autoimmune diseases, or you take medicine that suppresses immune function
- **Rare inherited conditions** — if you have a skin condition such as xeroderma pigmentosum, or certain hereditary breast and ovarian syndromes

> **"Never. Lose. Hope. Tomorrow could be the day you have been waiting for."**

How is melanoma treated?

Treatment for melanoma depends on the extent of the cancer known as its stage. Staging of melanoma happens twice: after biopsy and after surgery. The reason for two staging periods is because surgery often gives even more specific information than the original biopsy. This means the melanoma could be changed to a higher stage (upstaged) and treated differently at that point.

There are five stages of melanoma that range from stage 0 (in situ) to stage 4 (metastatic melanoma). For more detailed information on staging, read *Chapter 3: Staging for melanoma*.

The lower the number, the earlier the stage and the easier the melanoma is to treat with fewer treatments. The good news is that most melanomas are found in earlier stages. And even if melanoma is diagnosed at a later stage, many effective treatments are available.

Surgery is typically the primary treatment for earlier stages. To learn more, read *Chapter 5: Treatment for stages 0 to 2: Early stage.*

But for melanoma that has spread regionally, you might receive surgery along with other treatments like immunotherapy, intralesional talimogene laherparepvec (T-VEC) injections, targeted therapy, or radiation therapy. For more information, read *Chapter 6: Treatment for stage 3: Regional.*

Sometimes melanoma can return, which is called recurrence. It's treated based on its pathologic (after surgery) stage and if it has spread to another part of the body. In addition to surgery, you might receive treatment before it as well as after it. For more information on recurrence, read *Chapter 7: Treatment for recurrence.*

For stage 4 melanoma (metastatic), you might have a combination of systemic treatment, surgery, radiation, intralesional T-VEC injections, or supportive care. Read *Chapter 8: Treatment for stage 4: Metastatic disease* for more specific information.

What can you do to get the best care?

Advocate for yourself. You have an important role to play in your care. In fact, you're more likely to get the care you want by asking questions and making shared decisions with your care team.

The NCCN Guidelines for Patients will help you understand cancer care. With better understanding, you'll be more prepared to discuss your care with your team and share your concerns. Many people feel more satisfied when they play an active role in their care.

You may not know what to ask your care team. That's common. Each chapter in this book ends with an important section called *Questions to ask*. These suggested questions will help you get more information on all aspects of your care.

Take the next step and keep reading to learn what is the best care for you!

Why you should read this book

Making decisions about cancer care can be stressful. You may need to make tough decisions under pressure about complex choices.

The NCCN Guidelines for Patients are trusted by patients and providers. They clearly explain current care recommendations made by respected experts in the field. Recommendations are based on the latest research and practices at leading cancer centers.

Cancer care is not the same for everyone. By following expert recommendations for your situation, you are more likely to improve your care and have better outcomes as a result. Use this book as your guide to find the information you need to make important decisions.

2

Testing for melanoma

Treatment planning starts with testing. Accurate testing is needed to correctly identify the type of melanoma and to see if it has spread and how far. This chapter presents an overview of the tests you might receive and what to expect. Depending on the melanoma stage, you may not receive all of these tests.

Most melanomas are found in the early stages when they're easier to treat.

Basic health tests help your doctor detect diseases, including melanoma. Tests also help your care team assess the extent of the melanoma, which is called the cancer stage. You can read about melanoma cancer staging in more detail in the next chapter, *Chapter 3: Staging for melanoma.*

Medical history

A medical history is a record of all health issues and treatments you have had in your life. This information can help your doctor with treatment planning.

Be prepared to list any illnesses or injuries and when they happened. Bring a list of old and new medicines and any over-the-counter medicines, vitamins, or herbal supplements you take. Tell your doctor about any medical conditions or allergies you have. You should also tell your doctor if you have had any severe sunburns or other severe scarring in the past.

Your medical history also includes if you have had other types of skin cancers, such as basal cell skin cancer or squamous cell skin cancer. These are often less serious types of skin cancer.

More information on these types of skin cancer can be found in *NCCN Guidelines for Patients: Basal Cell Skin Cancer* and *NCCN Guidelines for Patients: Squamous Cell Skin Cancer*, available at NCCN.org/patientguidelines and on the NCCN Patient Guides for Cancer app.

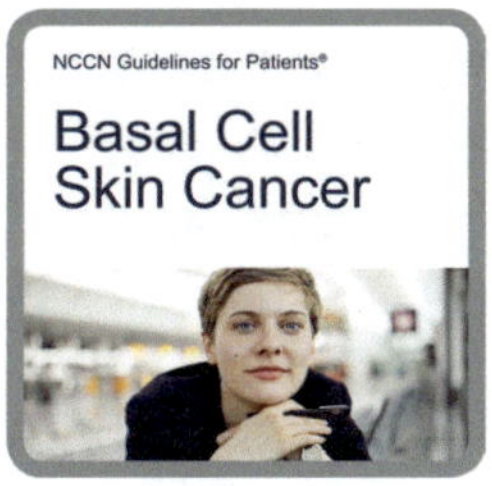

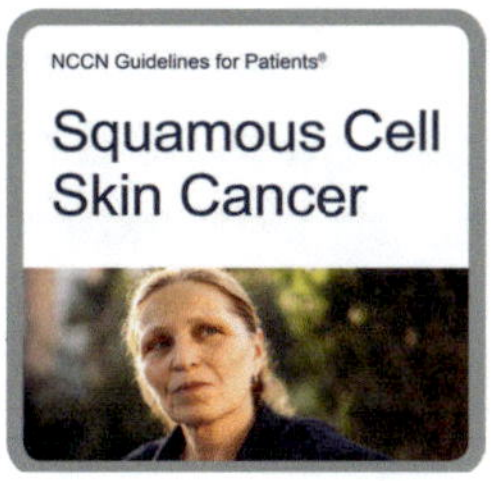

Family history

Your doctor will ask about the health history of family members who are blood relatives. This information is called a family history. Some cancers and other diseases can run in families. Ask family members about their health issues like heart disease, cancer, skin cancer, and diabetes, and at what age they were diagnosed. For more information on genetic risks, see *Chapter 9: Follow-up care.*

Physical exam

During a physical exam, a health care provider may:

- Check your temperature, blood pressure, pulse, and breathing rate
- Weigh you and measure your height
- Listen to your lungs and heart
- Look in your eyes, ears, nose, and throat
- Feel and apply pressure to parts of your body to see if organs are of normal size, are soft or hard, or cause pain when touched
- Feel for small structures called lymph nodes in your neck, underarm, and groin to see if they are bigger than normal

Skin exams

It's important to have an experienced health care provider, such as a dermatologist, give you a thorough skin exam. Skin exams are used for diagnosis, staging, and treatment planning. Expect a head-to-toe exam that includes a review of your:

- Head and scalp
- Face and mouth
- Eyes and eyelids
- Ears and earlobes
- Trunk, arms, and legs
- Hands and fingers
- Feet, toes, and toenails

Your provider will look for spots that are unusual and need to be examined more closely or monitored.

Not only does your skin protect your body, but it also tells doctors a lot about your health. Providers take your pulse and blood pressure through your skin. They notice if the skin feels warm, hot, or cool to the touch.

Skin exam

A health care provider may use a dermatoscope (a special magnifying lens and light source held near the skin) to see spots on the skin more clearly and with more detail.

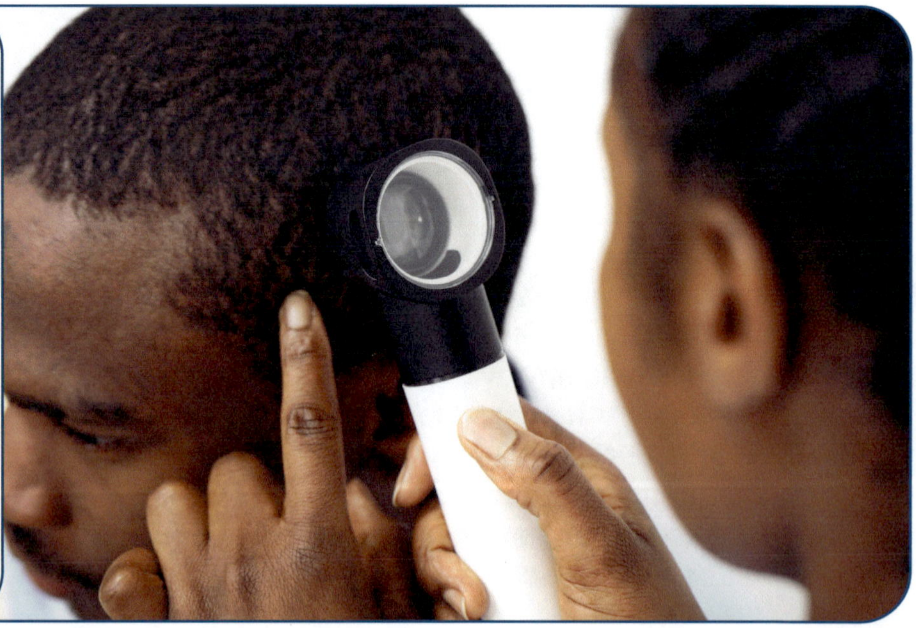

Lesions

Your provider will examine your skin for lesions (spots). A skin lesion is defined as a change in skin color or texture. Skin lesions can appear anywhere on your body. Lesions can be benign (not cancer) or cancer. Your doctor may use the ugly duckling or the ABCDE rule (mentioned in Chapter 9 of this book) to thoroughly review any marks or lesions on your skin or a specialized device called a dermatoscope. When a melanoma lesion is diagnosed, it is considered a cancerous tumor and will be referred that way throughout this book.

Skin color

Your skin color is mainly based on the amount of melanin in your skin. You know your skin better than anyone. Show your provider any changes or differences where your skin might look abnormal or different to you.

Guide 1 Common tests for melanoma
Medical and family history
Physical exam
Complete skin exam
Biopsy
Imaging tests
Biomarker tests
Blood tests (for monitoring)

Pay attention to moles

More than 50 moles on your body and the presence of large or unusual moles increases the risk of melanoma.

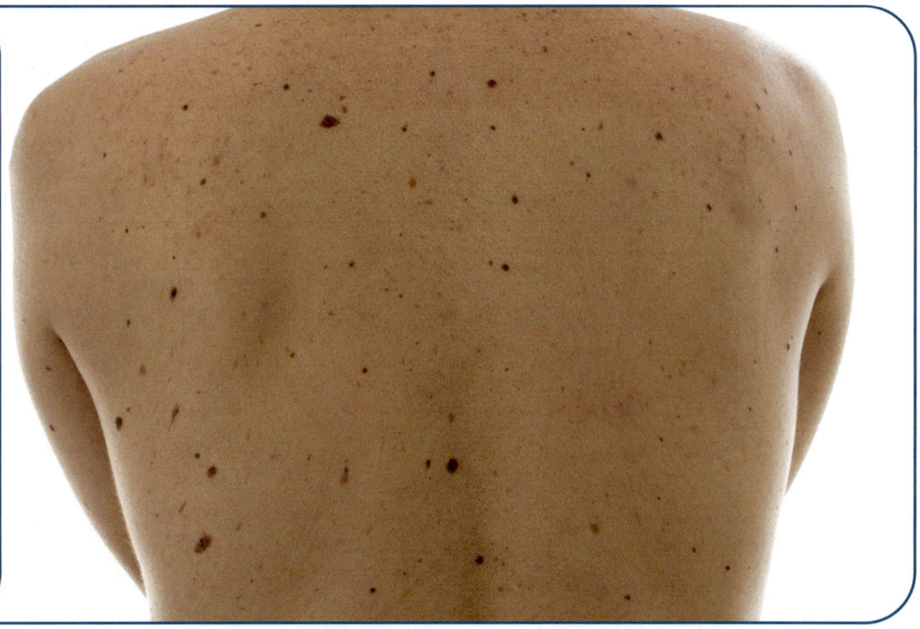

Biopsy tests

If you have a questionable skin lesion, part or all of it will be removed and sent to a laboratory to be looked at under a microscope by a pathologist. This is called a skin biopsy. A biopsy is needed to diagnose melanoma.

Skin biopsy types

Skin biopsies are done using a local anesthetic (numbing medicine), which is injected into the area with a very small needle. You will likely feel a small prick and a little stinging sensation as the medicine is injected, but you should not feel any pain during the biopsy.

You may also want to ask how the biopsy incision will be closed. Usually, it will be closed with stitches. Having a biopsy and incision usually means you will have a scar. You can ask your provider about the incision and the potential for scarring before you have the biopsy.

There are several ways to do a skin biopsy. The type of biopsy your provider chooses depends on its size and location, as well as other factors.

For the biopsy, all of your lesion or a sample of it will be removed and tested under the microscope to confirm melanoma.

A skin lesion biopsy can be partial (incisional) and not meant to completely remove the lesion or complete (excisional), removing all of the lesion.

A complete biopsy (excisional) is preferred for finding melanoma because it removes a larger area of skin than an incisional or partial biopsy. It can be done through an elliptical removal method, a punch method, or a deep shave

Skin punch biopsy

A small piece of skin and connective tissue are removed using a hand-held tool.

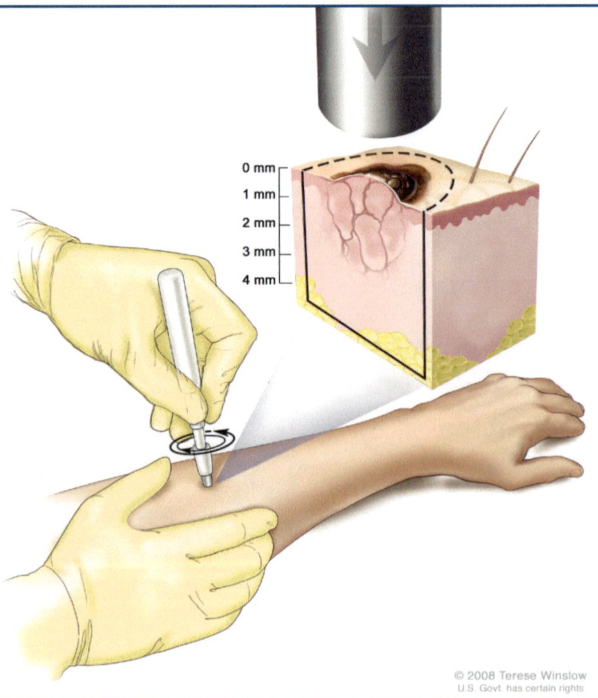

removal method (also called a saucerization biopsy).

Elliptical biopsy

An elliptical excisional biopsy removes an area of skin and underlying connective tissue, usually in the shape of a football. A rim of normal-looking tissue that surrounds the lesion will be removed, too. This normal-looking tissue is called the margin. This method requires stitches to close the wound.

Punch biopsy

For a punch biopsy of the skin, a small piece of skin and underlying connective tissue are removed using a handheld tool. A few stitches are then used to close the opening in the skin. One or more punch biopsies may be used on very large lesions, where a complete (excisional) biopsy isn't possible. This can help to avoid inaccurate pathology results.

Deep shave (saucerization) biopsy

A shave biopsy can be done either on the skin surface (superficial) or deeper. Superficial shave biopsies can be used when a lesion is likely not cancerous. They are generally not recommended when melanoma is suspected but may be useful for certain melanoma types (mainly, lentigo maligna) that are flat skin lesions.

But deep shave biopsies are used for most melanoma lesions to completely remove the suspicious skin lesion. This biopsy is also called a scoop biopsy or saucerization/shave removal. This type of biopsy uses a tool similar to a razor to remove the top layer of skin (epidermis) and part of the underlying layer (dermis). The sample is sent to the lab to be examined.

Lymph node biopsy

A lymph node might be biopsied if your provider suspects it has cancer cells. Lymph nodes are small, bean-shaped filters of the immune system. In normal circumstances, lymph nodes are usually too small to be seen or felt. But if a lymph node feels swollen, hard to the touch, or doesn't move when pushed (it feels fixed or immobile), it may be cancerous.

A lymph node biopsy can be done using a needle, which is preferred. It can also be done as a minor surgery to remove a lymph node, if it can't be biopsied with a needle.

Biopsy results

Your biopsy sample should be reviewed by a pathologist or preferably, by a dermatopathologist, who specializes in diagnosing skin disorders including melanoma and other skin tumors. This review is called a histopathology review. The pathologist will note the overall appearance and the size, shape, type of your cells, and other features. The melanoma will be given a stage based on this information and other factors. See the next chapter for more details on staging.

The pathologist or dermatopathologist will look for the following details:

Breslow thickness

The Breslow thickness or depth is used to measure in millimeters (mm) how far the melanoma has gone into the deeper layers of the skin (dermis). The deeper it goes, the more advanced the melanoma is. This is an important predictor and is used as part of melanoma staging to determine treatment.

Ulceration status

Ulceration refers to a breakdown of skin on top of the melanoma, like an open sore. An ulcerated melanoma is considered more serious because it has a greater risk of spreading. It is also used as part of melanoma staging.

Dermal mitotic rate

The dermal mitotic rate or mitotic rate (MR) is a measure of how fast cancer cells are growing and dividing in the dermis. The MR is measured by looking at the surgically removed tumor under a microscope. The number of cells that show mitoses (cells dividing) are counted.

The more the cells are dividing (higher mitotic count), the more likely they will invade the blood or lymph vessels and spread (metastasize) to other sites of the body.

Margin status (deep and peripheral)

The edge or border of the tissue removed in cancer surgery is called the margin. Margin status of a biopsy or excision specimen refers to whether the tumor is present at the deep (the base of the sample) or peripheral (side edges of the sample) margin.

The margin is described as negative or clear when the pathologist finds no cancer cells at the edge of the tissue, suggesting that all of the cancer has been removed.

The extent of the final surgical margin depends on how deep the melanoma is (the Breslow thickness). A wider excision of the melanoma is typically done after the initial biopsy, even if the margins are clear on initial biopsy.

Expect your doctor to remove the melanoma as well as a small amount of normal-looking skin around it. This margin helps to increase the chance that all cancerous cells will be removed. Speak to your provider about how much area around the tumor will be removed. They may draw it on your skin with a marker.

Microsatellitosis (present or absent)

Melanoma may metastasize (spread or travel) through your lymphatic system to the skin, subcutaneous (under the skin) tissues, and lymph nodes.

One way it can spread is through microsatellitosis (having microsatellite tumors). This refers to tiny tumor deposits that have spread to lymph vessels in the skin near the first melanoma tumor. Microsatellitosis can only be seen with a microscope.

These are different than satellite tumors, which are bigger and can be seen or felt. Satellite tumors are usually found within 2 centimeters (cm) from the melanoma site or scar and show as a nodule or bump. Any bumps beyond 2 cm from the melanoma are referred to as in-transit metastases.

Pure desmoplasia (if present)

Desmoplastic melanoma (DM) is a rare type of melanoma that is found most often on the head, neck, and shoulders. It occurs in 1 out of 25 people who have melanoma. It is divided into two categories: pure and mixed. Pure desmoplastic melanoma may be associated with a higher risk of local recurrence on the skin but has a lower risk of lymph node involvement. Mixed desmoplastic melanoma has a higher risk of spreading to nearby lymph nodes.

Lymphovascular or angiolymphatic invasion

Lymphovascular or angiolymphatic invasion refers to melanoma that has grown into (invaded) lymph vessels or blood vessels and is more aggressive (more likely to spread).

Neurotropism

Neurotropism or perineural invasion refers to melanoma growing around nerves in the skin or within nerves (called intraneural invasion). It is most often seen in desmoplastic melanoma and has a higher tendency to recur on the skin or nearby.

For a list of what factors will be considered when pathologists analyze biopsies, **see Guide 2.** Your pathologist or dermatopathologist might also use specific immunohistochemical stains or molecular tests to detect markers on melanoma cells.

Guide 2 Factors examined in the biopsy
Breslow thickness (how deep the melanoma tumor has grown into the skin)
Ulceration status (if there are breaks on the skin)
Dermal mitotic rate (a measure of how fast cancer cells grow)
Deep and peripheral margin status (if the area around the tumor is free from cancer)
Microsatellitosis (if there are small satellite lesions that aren't part of the primary lesion)
Pure desmoplasia (if there is fibrous tissue within a tumor)
Lymphovascular or angiolymphatic invasion (if cancer is in lymph nodes or fluid)
Neurotropism (invasion in, around, and through peripheral nerves)

Imaging (radiology) tests

Imaging tests take pictures (images) of the inside of your body. These tests are sometimes used for cancer staging or to check symptoms. However, not everyone needs imaging, especially for the early stages of melanoma.

For most of these testing scans, contrast materials will be used. Contrast materials are substances that help certain areas in the body stand out. They are used to make the pictures clearer. Contrast materials are not permanent and will leave the body in your urine. They will usually be given orally (by mouth) or intravenously (injected with a needle through the vein), which is called an IV contrast.

Most scans will be performed with IV contrast unless it is unsafe for you. This means it could cause a bad reaction if you have certain allergies or conditions or take certain medications. It is important to tell your doctors if you ever had an allergic reaction to contrast.

After imaging, a radiologist, an expert in interpreting test images, will write a report and send this report to your provider. Your test results will be discussed with you. The general types of imaging tests include:

CT scan

A computed tomography (CT or CAT) scan is a computerized x-ray machine. It takes many pictures (x-rays) from different angles of the same body part. Pictures are merged to form a 3D image.

MRI scan

A magnetic resonance imaging (MRI) scan uses strong magnets and radio waves to take digital pictures of the inside of the body. It does not use x-rays.

CT machine

A CT machine is large and has a tunnel in the middle. During the test, you will lie on a table that moves slowly through the tunnel.

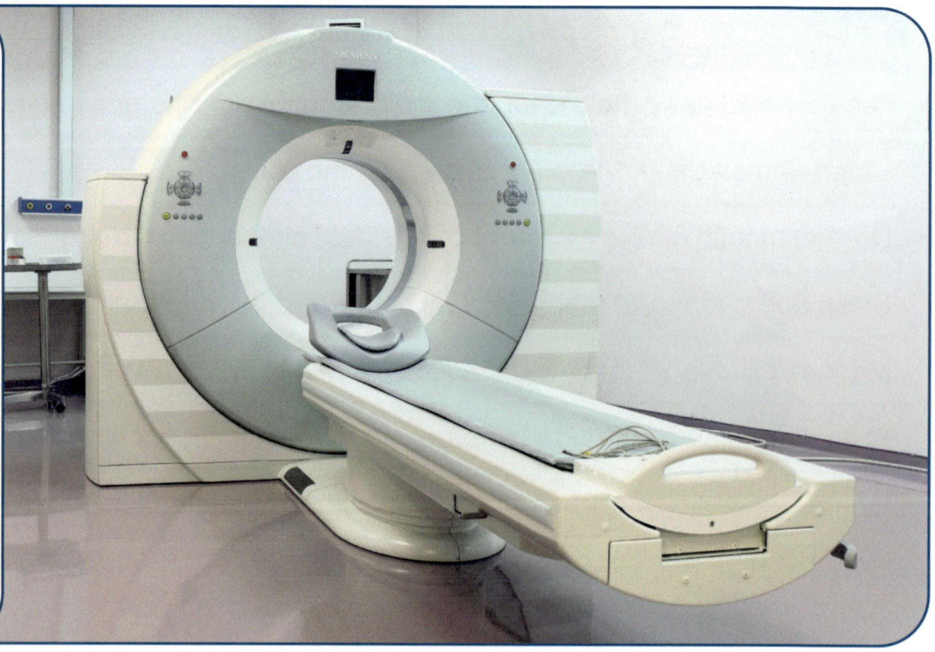

PET scan

A positron emission tomography (PET) scan uses a radioactive drug called a tracer. A tracer is injected into a vein (through an IV). The needle is most often inserted on the inside of your elbow. You may need to wait for the tracer to be absorbed by your body, which takes about 1 hour.

Once inside the body, the tracer will travel and collect in organs and tissues. The tracer is attached to a substance that your cells and tissues use for energy or food. Cancer cells use more of this substance than non-cancer cells.

Cancer cells show up as bright spots on PET scans. Not all bright spots are cancer. It is normal for the brain, heart, kidneys, and bladder to be bright on a PET scan since they require a lot of food or energy. When a PET scan is combined with CT, it is called a PET/CT scan, and they are almost always used together.

Ultrasound

Ultrasound uses sound waves to make pictures of areas inside of the body. Your provider might order a nodal basin ultrasound before removing lymph nodes. This is to get a clearer picture of the area before the lymph node removal.

Biomarker testing is usually done in advanced stages (stage 3 and stage 4) of melanoma. But not everyone with melanoma in those stages will need this type of testing.

Uses for biomarker testing

Biomarker or molecular testing can be used in the following instances:

- To help diagnose cancer
- To help determine your prognosis or see how advanced your cancer is, especially the risk of metastasis (how likely it is to spread)
- To find genetic mutations that happen after birth that can be treated with a targeted therapy or an immune therapy
- To help you and your care team with treatment planning

Biomarker tests

Biomarkers are specific features of cancer cells. Biomarkers can include proteins made in response to cancer and/or reflect changes (mutations) in the DNA of cancer cells. A mutation might cause a gene to create a protein and keep making it. This can lead to the development of a tumor.

Testing on biomarkers involves studying a piece of tumor tissue in a lab or testing a blood sample (also called a liquid biopsy). Other names for biomarker testing include molecular testing, tumor profiling, genomic testing, tumor gene testing, next-generation sequencing, and mutation testing.

Immunohistochemistry (IHC) is a common and quick lab test of biomarkers that involves adding a chemical marker to immune cells. The cells are then studied under a microscope. IHC might be used to see if cancer has spread, or to look for mutations such as *BRAF* or PD-L1 proteins. It may also be used to help tell the difference between different types of cancer.

Biomarker testing is used to learn whether the cancer has any targetable changes to help guide your treatment. The results of the biomarker testing can also be used to determine whether you meet criteria for joining certain clinical trials.

BRAF mutations

BRAF is a gene involved with controlling normal cell growth. But when a *BRAF* gene has mutated (changed), it can cause melanoma to grow more aggressively. A *BRAF* mutation is found in at least half of people who have melanoma in the skin.

It is helpful if the *BRAF* gene mutation is found before treatment for advanced disease. Health care providers can use targeted therapy to inhibit (stop) the *BRAF* gene mutation from continuing to grow the cancer.

If IHC detects a *BRAF* V600E mutation, targeted therapy or immunotherapy may be a treatment option, if needed.

If IHC does not detect a *BRAF* V600E mutation, a more specialized test like polymerase chain reaction (PCR) or next generation sequencing (NGS) may be used. These tests may also detect *BRAF* V600K and other mutations like *NRAS* and *KIT*.

Blood tests

Blood tests check for signs of disease and how well organs are working. They use a sample of your blood, which is removed through a needle placed into your vein.

Blood tests are not used to diagnose melanoma or monitor early melanomas. However, they may be done before or during treatment, especially for more advanced melanomas.

Tests that your provider may request include:

Lactate dehydrogenase — Lactate dehydrogenase (LDH) is a protein found in most cells. Dying cells release LDH into blood. A high LDH level is a sign that the melanoma may have spread to other parts of the body and may be harder to treat. This blood test may be done if your care provider suspects the cancer has spread to distant sites (called stage 4 or metastatic cancer).

Other blood tests — Other blood tests are not regularly done before starting treatment. But they may be done to plan surgical treatment. If you have advanced melanoma, these tests might be done to define whether the bone marrow, liver, and kidneys are working before and during treatment. This may include a complete blood count (CBC) or comprehensive metabolic panel (CMP). A CMP can check liver and kidney health, blood glucose, protein levels, fluid and electrolytes, and metabolism.

Understanding test results

The results of your physical exam, skin biopsy, and possible imaging scans will guide your treatment plan. It's important you understand what these tests mean. Don't hesitate to ask your care team questions.

Keep these other tips in mind:

- Bring someone with you to your appointments, if possible.
- Write down questions before your appointments and take notes during clinic visits.
- Get copies of blood tests, imaging results, and reports about the specific type of cancer you have.
- Sign up for the patient portal. If your provider offers an online patient portal, ask about opening an account. Once on the portal, you can get test results as soon as they're ready, in most cases.
- Organize your papers. Create files for insurance forms, medical records, and test results. You can do the same on your computer, if you have one.

Positive vs. Negative Results
The truth of what they mean

It might seem confusing and like the opposite of what you'd think at first. But it's important to know that when you hear of a **positive** result in cancer testing, it means that the **cancer was found**. When you hear of a **negative** result, that means the **cancer was not found**.

What's next

This chapter gave an overview of the different types of tests, from skin exams and genetic tests to imaging, that are used to diagnose melanoma. Now that you know the kinds of tests you might have, read the next chapter on the variety of treatments available. To find out more specifically how the melanoma might be treated, read about it in the stage-specific chapters.

Key points

- Basic health tests help your care team assess the extent (cancer stage) of the melanoma.
- A medical history is a record of all health issues and treatments you have had in your life including other cancers.
- A head-to-toe skin exam should include a review of the scalp, face, mouth, eyes and eyelids, ears, trunk and extremities, hands, fingers, feet, toes, and toenails. This includes examining your skin for lesions (spots).
- A melanoma diagnosis is primarily based on the results of a skin biopsy. If you have an unusual lesion, it will be removed and sent to a lab to be examined.
- Imaging tests take pictures of the inside of your body, which are examined to look for cancer. Not everyone with melanoma needs imaging tests.
- Biomarker or molecular tests look for certain genes, proteins, or other molecules in a sample of tissue, blood, or other bodily fluid. These tests are sometimes used to help diagnose melanoma, and to stage and treat it.
- Blood tests may be done if you have surgery, if your care provider suspects the cancer has spread, or if you are taking systemic treatment for melanoma.

Questions to ask

- Why did I get this specific test?
- Do the tests have any risks?
- Do I need to do anything to prepare for testing?
- Do I need other tests to confirm my diagnosis?
- How much scarring will there be from the biopsy?

“

You can only control what you can control. Let go of anything that is not serving you well and stay present in the moment."

3 Staging for melanoma

A cancer stage is a way to describe the extent of the cancer at the time you are first diagnosed. Staging is needed to make treatment decisions, and it happens twice with melanoma: after biopsy and after surgery. Understanding the melanoma stage is very important so don't hesitate to ask your care team questions.

The thickness of a melanoma tumor is measured in millimeters (mm). The tip of a pencil is about 1 mm thick.

TNM staging

The American Joint Committee on Cancer (AJCC) TNM staging system is widely used to stage melanoma. In this system, the letters T (tumor), N (node or lymph node status), and M (metastasis or spread) describe different areas of cancer growth. The TNM stages will be combined to assign the cancer stage group.

- **Tumor depth (T)** refers to the thickness of the primary tumor and whether the tumor has broken through the skin like an open sore (this is called ulceration). Tumor depth is measured in millimeters (mm). There are five tumor designations (Tis, T1, T2, T3 and T4). See figure.
- **Lymph node status (N)** describes whether the cancer has spread nearby (regionally) through small tubes called lymph vessels or to small bean-shaped structures (in the neck, armpits, or groin) called lymph nodes. It also includes in-transit, satellite, and/or microsatellite tumors. For more information on these tumors, see *Chapter 6: Treatment for stage 3: Regional*.
- **Metastasis (M)** describes whether the cancer has spread to parts of the body far away from the primary tumor, like internal organs and distant lymph nodes. This tends to be lungs, liver, bones, brain, and gastrointestinal (GI) tract. There are only two designations for metastasis: either the cancer has spread to distant areas (M1), or it has not (M0). For more information on metastatic melanoma, see *Chapter 8, Treatment for stage 4: Metastatic disease.*

There are 5 stages of melanoma, including stage 0. Doctors may write the later stages (1 through 4) as Roman numerals: stages I, II, III, and IV.

Based on cancer test results described in Chapter 2, your doctor will assign a melanoma stage (0, 1, 2, 3, or 4). Many times, that stage will be accompanied by a letter (A, B, C, or D).

The higher the stage, the thicker the tumor or the more the cancer has spread.

Clinical vs. pathological

With melanoma, you will be staged twice. The first time is called clinical staging. The second time is called pathological staging.

- **Clinical staging** happens after the biopsy. This is when you find out you have a diagnosis of melanoma and what stage it is.
- **Pathological staging** happens after you have surgery to remove the tumor and surrounding area (and nearby lymph nodes, if needed) to see how advanced the cancer is. The cancer may have changed from the clinical stage or the additional information from the surgery might alter the stage. This is especially true when a sentinel lymph node biopsy is done and finds melanoma microscopically in nearby lymph nodes.

While the clinical stage helps guide treatment, the pathological stage is more accurate and specific. The pathological stage involves more information from the surgery to clarify your diagnosis and guide further treatment.

Breslow thickness: What is it?

In your pathology report you might see Breslow depth or thickness mentioned. This is the measurement in millimeters (mm) of how deep or thick the melanoma tumor is.

Stages of melanoma

The TNM classification of malignant tumors reflecting tumor thickness

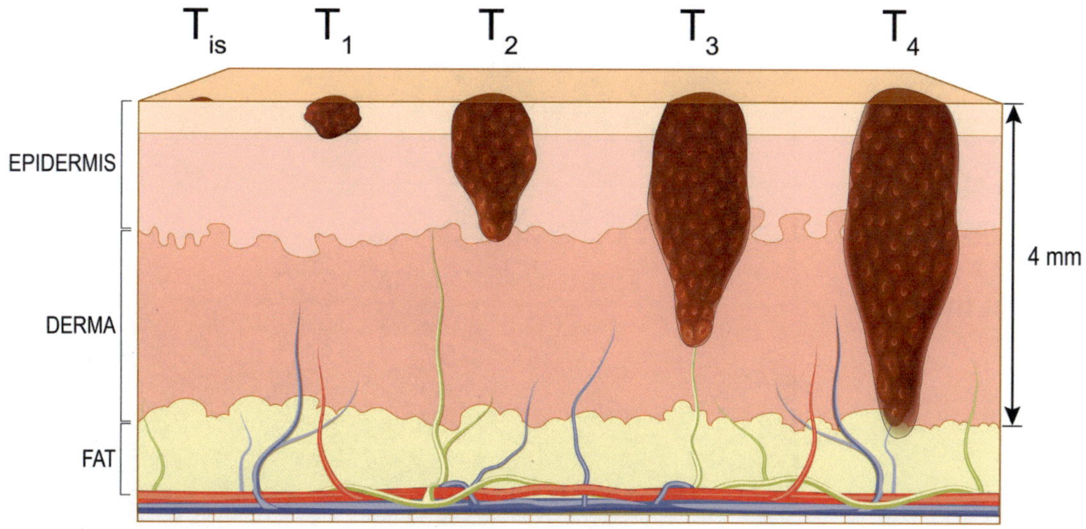

A summary of stages

Because it might be challenging to follow the clinical and pathological stages on their own, they are summarized below and described in more detail in the stage-specific chapters.

In general, **stage 0, stage 1, and stage 2 melanoma** are early cancers in the skin that are not known to have spread elsewhere. Surgery is the most common treatment. For more detailed information on early-stage melanoma, see *Chapter 5: Treatment for stages 0 to 2: Early stage.*

Stage 3 melanoma has spread but is considered regional. Once the tumor is considered stage 3, it involves the lymph nodes and lymphatic vessels and after surgery, it is broken down into four pathological stages (3A, 3B, 3C, and 3D). For more detailed information on stage 3 melanoma, see *Chapter 6: Treatment for stage 3: Regional.*

Stage 4 melanoma is cancer that has spread (metastasized) to distant areas of the body such as the lungs, liver, brain, bones or GI tract. For more detailed information on stage 4 melanoma, see *Chapter 8: Treatment for stage 4: Metastatic disease.*

If you have any questions, be sure to ask your provider to explain the melanoma in a way that you can best understand it.

What's next

Now that you have learned about how and why melanoma is staged, the next step is treatment. The following chapter is about all the different types of treatment for melanoma. Keep in mind that it's an overview and no one will receive every treatment. When you find out the melanoma's stage, you can read all about the treatment for it in the stage-specific treatment chapters that follow.

While a diagnosis of melanoma can be scary, many advances in treatment have been made in the past decade.

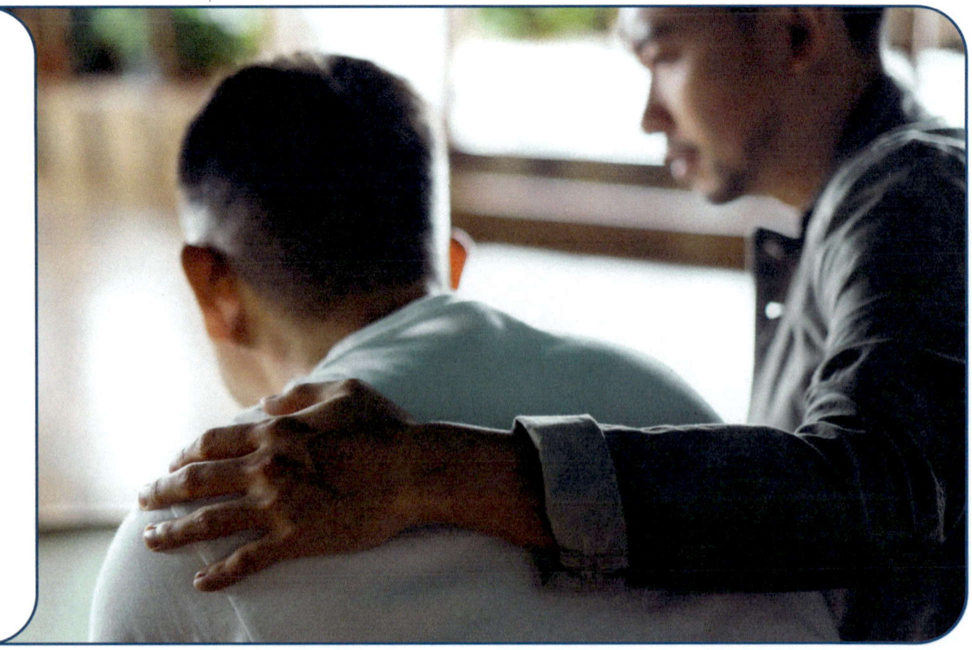

Key points

- Staging for melanoma is needed to make appropriate treatment choices.
- Staging helps describe the depth of the tumor, whether any lymph nodes are involved, and whether or not the melanoma has spread (metastasized).
- You will be staged for cancer twice: after biopsy (clinical stage) and after surgery (pathological stage).
- The clinical stage helps guide treatment, but the pathological stage is more accurate.
- Stage 0 through stage 2 are considered early stage cancer.
- Stage 3 melanoma has spread only to nearby tissues, so it is called regional.
- Stage 4 melanoma refers to cancer that has spread (metastasized) to distant areas of the body.

Questions to ask

- What stage is the melanoma at biopsy?
- When will I have surgery?
- Where will I have surgery?
- Are the lymph nodes involved?
- What other health professionals will be a part of my care team?

4
Treatment overview

This chapter describes the kinds of treatments you may receive for melanoma. It's important to know that not everyone will receive the same treatment. Treatment for melanoma is based on its stage and location. For more information on your stage, follow the stage-specific chapters.

Who is on your care team?

After being diagnosed, knowing what to do next can be overwhelming and confusing. But you have a care team to help. Aside from your primary care provider (such as your family doctor), there are several medical professionals who will help you make decisions about your treatment and supportive care.

Depending on your diagnosis, your care team might include the following specialists.

Doctors who treat cancer

Dermatologists diagnose and treat skin conditions, including skin cancer. They also do skin exams and help you learn how to do them on your own. Some dermatologists also perform surgery.

Surgical oncologists are trained to diagnose and surgically treat and remove cancerous tumors.

Medical oncologists specialize in prescribing cancer drugs. They are trained to diagnose and treat cancer using special medicines that may be taken by mouth or given through a vein (intravenously).

Radiation oncologists are trained to use different types of radiation to destroy cancerous cells while keeping other cells healthy.

Pathologists are trained to study tissue and cells removed during a biopsy under a microscope to determine the diagnosis and stage of a tumor. Dermatopathologists are experts in skin pathology.

Plastic surgeons reconstruct, restore, and repair body parts. They may be needed to close a wound after surgery, especially if it involves deeper tissue.

Head and neck surgeons treat diseases (both cancerous and noncancerous) of the head and neck.

Guide 3 Common treatments for melanoma
Surgery
Targeted therapy
Immunotherapy
Radiation therapy
Clinical trials

Other health professionals

Oncology nurses provide hands-on care, like giving systemic therapy, managing your care plan, answering questions, and helping you cope with side effects. Sometimes these experts are called nurse navigators.

Pharmacists are trained to prepare and give out medicine and teach about their proper use and any side effects. Some pharmacists specifically work with people with cancer.

Geneticists study how traits are passed down from parents to children through genes. They are trained to diagnose and treat genetic disorders and counsel people and families at risk.

Nutritionists and dietitians help guide you on what foods are most suitable for your diagnosis and treatment.

Palliative care nurses help provide an extra layer of support with the cancer-related symptoms.

Psychologists and psychiatrists can help you manage mental health issues such as depression, anxiety, or other conditions that can affect how you feel during treatment.

Social workers help people solve and cope with problems in their everyday lives while they are undergoing treatment.

Some members of your care team will be with you throughout your treatment and beyond, while others will be there for parts of it.

You know your body better than anyone. Help other team members understand:

- How you feel
- What you need
- What is working and what isn't
- Your goals for treatment

Keep a list of names and contact information for each member of your team. Add it to your smartphone, too, if you have one. Hang the list in an obvious place where anyone can access it in an emergency.

This will make it easier for you and anyone else who is involved in your care to know who to contact with questions or concerns.

Surgery

Surgery is an operation or procedure to remove cancer from the body. The type of surgery depends on the size, number, and location of the cancer. Surgery is the primary treatment for most melanomas.

A person diagnosed with melanoma should expect to have surgery following the skin biopsy.

The goal of surgery for a primary melanoma tumor is to remove all the cancer from your body. For melanomas that have a low risk of spread, surgery may be the only treatment needed. There are different types of surgery used for melanoma.

Wide excision

A wide excision surgery removes the melanoma tumor as well as normal tissue surrounding it (the surgical margin). The surgical margin is measured in centimeters (cm). The size to be removed depends on the thickness of the primary tumor (**see Guide 4**).

A wide excision may be done in a doctor's office, surgical center, or hospital (operating room).

You may receive local anesthesia before the surgery. Local anesthesia is medicine that numbs a small area of the body to minimize pain during the surgery. Most stage 0 and stage 1 melanomas are treated under local anesthesia.

For deeper or more advanced melanomas that require lymph node biopsy (described ahead) or more extensive surgery, general anesthesia may be used. You will be fully asleep during the surgery.

A wide excision is done even if the melanoma tumor was removed by biopsy. A wide excision will also remove nearby microsatellites and lymph vessels in the skin because they could contain additional tumor cells and any nearby microsatellites.

A wide excision is often cut as an ellipse (football shape), which allows the wound to heal as a flat line. The surgical margin will be cut based on the thickness of the melanoma tumor.

Side effects of wide excision

Side effects of wide excision surgery may include pain, swelling, numbness and/or scarring. Pain and swelling are usually temporary and should only last for a few weeks after surgery. Scars can be a lasting

Guide 4
Surgical margin guidelines for wide excision for melanoma

If your tumor thickness is:	The recommended surgical margin is:
In situ	0.5 to 1 cm
Less than 1 mm	1 cm
Greater than 1 to 2 mm	1 to 2 cm
Greater than 2 to 4 mm	2 cm
Greater than 4 mm	2 cm

result of surgery. Talk to your doctor if you are concerned about scars due to the surgery.

Following the surgery, a skin graft might be recommended for larger incisions. A skin graft is when a surgeon takes skin from another part of your body and uses it to cover the wound.

Skin grafts are surgeries that can be performed in the clinic or hospital. Most larger skin grafts involve sedation (giving medicine to help relax you) or general anesthesia, which means you'll be asleep throughout the procedure and won't feel any pain.

Sometimes, rotational "flaps" of tissue may be used to cover the wound so you can avoid a skin graft. A skin flap is a type of wound closure that takes skin from an area close to a wound and layers it to fill the removal of a skin lesion. Talk to your doctor about your options and how you can expect to heal after wide excision surgery.

Sentinel lymph node biopsy

A sentinel lymph node is the first lymph node where cancer cells most likely spread from a primary tumor on the skin. Sometimes there is more than one sentinel lymph node identified or multiple lymph node basins involved, like both armpit areas. The lymph node basin is the area of lymph nodes where lymph from the tumor drains.

A sentinel lymph node biopsy (SLNB) is a surgery that removes one or more lymph nodes to examine for any cancer cells. These nodes will be checked by a pathologist in a lab. (Most people with melanoma have an SLNB at the same time as wide excision surgery.)

The results will be used to stage the cancer and plan treatment.

To locate the sentinel lymph node(s), your surgeon or the radiology team will inject a radioactive substance (and in some cases, a blue-colored dye) into your skin near the

Wide excision

A wide excision surgery removes the melanoma tumor as well as some normal-looking tissue surrounding it.

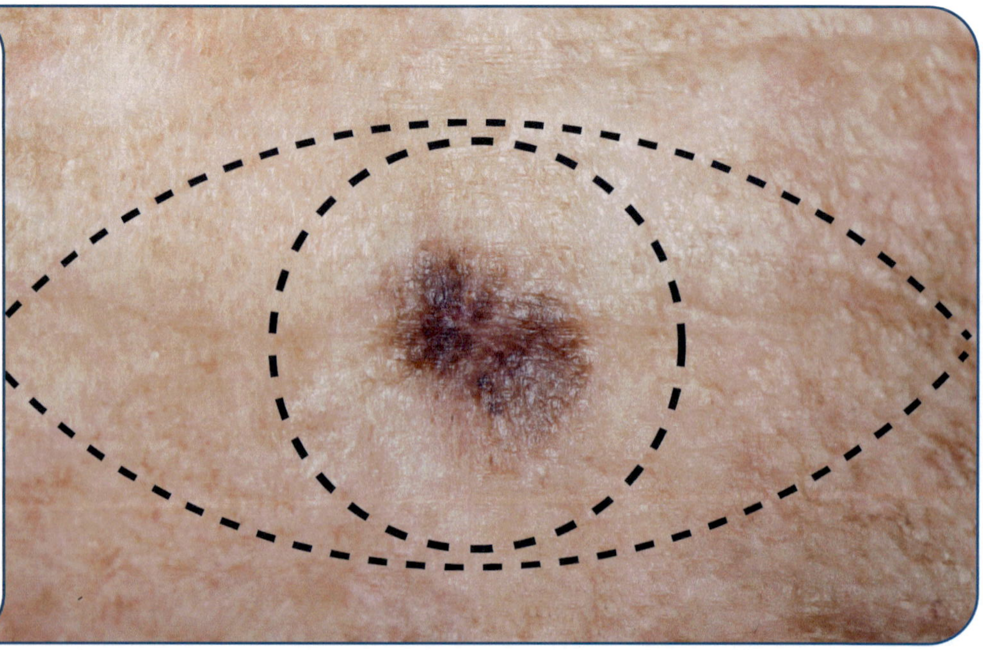

tumor. The substance will drain into the sentinel lymph nodes. Your surgeon will identify the sentinel lymph nodes using a device and remove them through a small cut in your skin. This procedure is typically done under general anesthesia.

Side effects of SLNB

You could experience some side effects after an SLNB, including numbness, pain, or bruising.

You could also develop a seroma, which is a pocket of clear fluid in the lymph node basin. A seroma usually goes away on its own but sometimes may need to be drained with a needle.

Your doctor or care team should discuss with you the possible risks and benefits of an SLNB before you have the surgery.

Lymph node dissection

A lymph node dissection is a surgical procedure where lymph nodes are removed and checked for cancer. The procedure may be done if the cancer has spread to the lymph node basin. This is not often done if there is cancer only in sentinel lymph node(s). A lymph node dissection removes nodes to prevent disease from coming back or spreading elsewhere. This surgery is done under general anesthesia.

Complete (also known as completion) lymph node dissection (CLND) refers to a dissection done after tiny amounts of cancer are found in the SLNB. It is not often performed after SLNB for most people, and nodal ultrasound or other imaging tests can be used instead to monitor the lymph nodes.

Lymph node dissection is generally recommended for advanced melanomas with enlarged lymph nodes found on clinical exam or imaging. Or it's done for nodes that have grown over time and have shown to contain melanoma.

Therapeutic lymph node dissection (TLND) is often combined with systemic drug therapy before surgery that shrinks the

Lymph nodes

There are hundreds of small bean-shaped structures throughout the human body called lymph nodes. Lymph nodes catch and filter out foreign particles and harmful cells, including cancer cells.

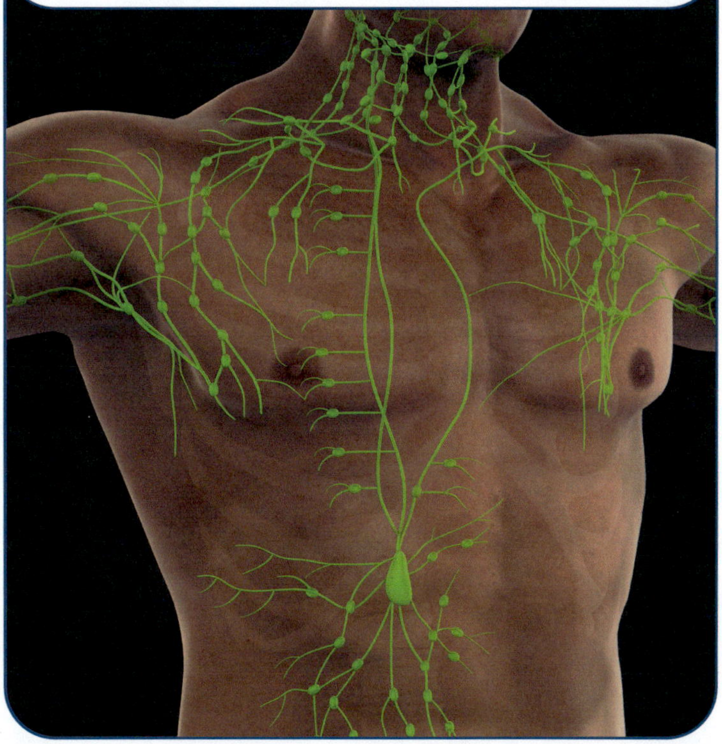

tumor (neoadjuvant therapy) or after surgery (adjuvant therapy).

Common side effects of TLND include pain, numbness, limited movement (of arms or legs), and lymphedema. Lymphedema is the most serious side effect of lymph node surgery because it causes swelling and discomfort in body parts, most commonly in the arms or legs. It is treated with compression therapy and/or physical therapy.

More information about managing lymphedema can be found in *NCCN Guidelines for Patients: Survivorship Care for Cancer-Related Late and Long-Term Effects,* available at NCCN.org/patientguidelines and on the NCCN Patient Guides for Cancer app

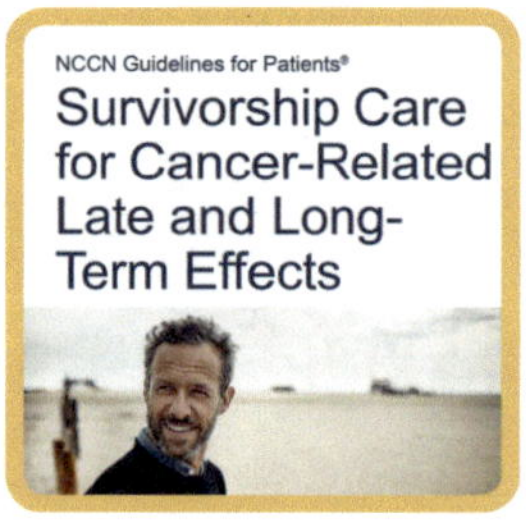

Targeted therapy

Targeted therapy drugs are designed to target and attack specific cancer cells. For melanoma, these drugs target the activity of a specific or unique feature of melanoma cells and interfere with how those cancer cells grow.

Cancer growth inhibitors

Cancer growth inhibitors (or blockers) are a type of targeted therapy that stops cancer cells from growing. Our bodies make chemicals called growth factors that control cell growth.

Cancer growth blockers work by blocking the growth factors that trigger cancer cells to

Order of Treatments

Most people with melanoma will receive more than one type of treatment. This is an overview of the order of treatments and what they do.

Neoadjuvant (before) treatment is given to shrink the tumor before primary treatment (surgery). This might make surgery possible for some challenging melanoma tumors.

Primary treatment is the main treatment given to rid the body of cancer. Surgery is usually the main treatment when the tumor can be removed, often in early stage melanoma.

- **First-line treatment** is the first set of cancer drugs given.
- **Second-line treatment** is the next set of cancer drugs given if the first-line treatment hasn't worked.

Adjuvant (after) treatment is given after primary treatment to rid the body of any cancer cells left behind from surgery. It is also used when the risk of cancer returning (recurrence) is felt to be high.

Talk with your doctor about your treatment plan and what it means for your stage of melanoma.

divide and grow. They are often taken orally (by mouth) and can be taken at home.

There are several types of cancer growth inhibitors, including:

- **BRAF inhibitors:** When a *BRAF* gene mutates, it gives faulty instructions to proteins that can help cancer cells grow. BRAF inhibitors are drugs that directly attack these proteins. They can shrink or slow the growth of tumors in melanoma that has spread or can't be removed completely. Types of BRAF inhibitors include vemurafenib (Zelboraf), dabrafenib (Tafinlar), and encorafenib (Braftovi).
- **MEK inhibitors:** MEK is a protein that is activated when the *BRAF* gene mutates and causes melanoma cancer cells to grow. Drugs known as MEK inhibitors target and attack the MEK protein. They are often used in combination with BRAF inhibitors. The MEK inhibitors include trametinib (Mekinist), cobimetinib (Cotellic), and binimetinib (Mektovi).
- **KIT inhibitors:** Mutations in the *KIT* gene can cause some rarer melanomas to develop, like those on the palms, soles, or under nail beds. Types of KIT inhibitors include imatinib (Gleevec), dasatinib (Sprycel), and nilotinib (Tasigna).

In most cases, BRAF inhibitors are combined with MEK inhibitors to treat melanomas that have mutations in the *BRAF* genes. These combinations include:

- Dabrafenib (Tafinlar) and trametinib (Mekinist)
- Encorafenib (Braftovi) and binimetinib (Mektovi)
- Vemurafenib (Zelboraf) and cobimetinib (Cotellic)

From the time of diagnosis, ask your doctor about participating in a clinical trial of a melanoma treatment. Clinical trials can be an option at any stage of disease.

BRAF and MEK inhibitors can cause non-melanoma skin cell cancers, photosensitivity (being sensitive to sunlight), other skin reactions, and many possible systemic side effects, including rash, nausea, diarrhea, loss of appetite, and fatigue. In some cases, side effects can be severe and even life-threatening, so tell your doctor if you have any of them.

If you develop a reaction on your skin (rash, itching, swelling) after you have any of the systemic therapies listed above, it is recommended that you see a dermatologist regularly for treatment.

Immunotherapy

The immune system is the body's defense against infection and disease. Immunotherapy is a treatment that uses the immune system to kill cancer cells.

Your immune system can tell the difference between normal cells in the body and those it sees as foreign, like germs and cancer cells. And for the most part, it will do its job to fight the foreign cells but not the normal cells.

T cells are a key part of the immune system. T cells that kill infected cells and cancer cells are called cytotoxic or killer T cells.

But sometimes the proteins on tumor cells bind with T-cell proteins, which prevents the T cells from killing the tumor cells. These tumor cell proteins are called immune checkpoint proteins. PD-L1 is a tumor cell checkpoint protein that can bind with PD-1 checkpoint protein on T-cells.

Checkpoint inhibitors

Immune checkpoint inhibitors are a type of immunotherapy. They work by blocking the proteins from binding, which then frees the T cells to kill the tumor cells.

Checkpoint inhibitors are slowly injected into a vein (infusion). It may take up to 30 to 60 minutes to get the full dose. Infusions are usually given every few weeks. The number of weeks between treatments can depend on the type of inhibitor used.

A new form of checkpoint inhibitor is available that can be injected under the skin (subcutaneously). It can be given every 2 weeks or every 4 weeks. It's a combination of nivolumab and hyaluronidase-nvhy (known as Opdivo Qvantig). The injectable form can be used instead of the IV nivolumab, but not in combination with ipilimumab.

Examples of checkpoint inhibitors that are used to treat melanoma include:

- Pembrolizumab (Keytruda)
- Nivolumab (Opdivo)

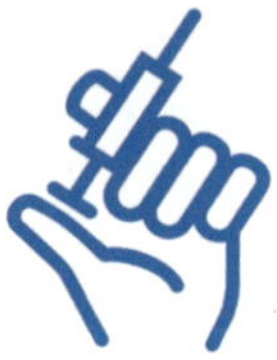

Are there vaccines that treat melanoma?

There are vaccines that can treat melanoma. But unlike vaccines for flu, pneumonia, and other illnesses, melanoma vaccines don't prevent melanoma. Instead, melanoma vaccines can be used to stop cancer from returning if you already had surgery to remove tumors. Vaccine therapies for melanoma are often tested in clinical trials. Vaccines for melanoma can be given either through **systemic** or **local** treatment.

Systemic treatment is usually given through drugs that release antigens through the bloodstream to boost the body's immune system so it can fight cancer. These drugs target the parts of melanoma cells that make them different from normal cells. They work differently from chemotherapy drugs, which attack both normal and cancer cells.

Local treatment directs antigens to a specific organ or area of the body, such as an abnormal growth on the skin. After surgery, these treatments could include forms of topical therapy (medicine in a lotion or cream that is applied directly to the skin).

- Nivolumab and hyaluronidase-nvhy (Opdivo Qvantig)
- Ipilimumab (Yervoy)
- Atezolizumab (Tecentriq)
- Nivolumab and relatlimab-rmbw (Opdualag)

Immunotherapy can be given alone or combined with other types of treatment. In some cases, a combination of an immunotherapy with another immunotherapy or an immunotherapy with a targeted therapy is recommended for treatment. Two examples of combinations are:

- Nivolumab* and ipilimumab
  - **Nivolumab and hyaluronidase injectable cannot be used in combination with ipilimumab*
- Nivolumab and relatlimab-rmbw

Checkpoint inhibitors can cause immune-related side effects, including rash, diarrhea, shortness of breath, headache, and abnormal thyroid function. These side effects can occur during or after treatment and in some cases be lifelong.

For more information, see *NCCN Guidelines for Patients: Immunotherapy Side Effects* at NCCN.org/patientguidelines and on the NCCN Patient Guides for Cancer app.

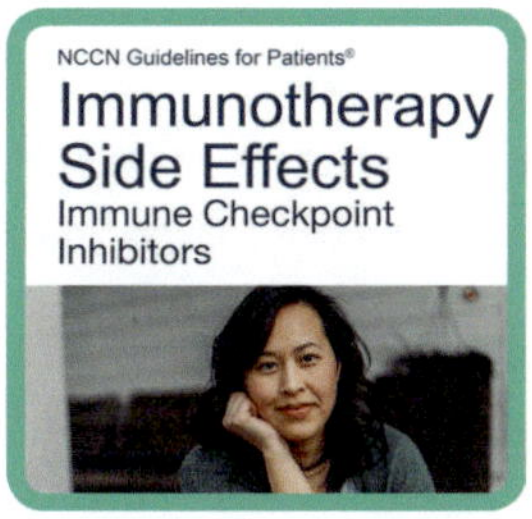

IL-2

Interleukin 2 (IL-2, Proleukin) is an immunotherapy that can be slowly injected into a vein (infusion) or directly into the cancer tumor. IL-2 is a group of proteins made by white blood cells and other cells that are responsible for increasing immune response. The therapy works by supercharging the immune system to target and kill cancer cells.

Side effects of IL-2 can include fever, chills, decrease in blood pressure, muscle stiffness, diarrhea, dizziness, tiredness, headache, weight gain, nausea, vomiting, and loss of appetite.

IL-2 can also be used with TIL (tumor-infiltrating lymphocytes) therapy.

T-VEC

Talimogene laherparepvec (T-VEC) (Imlygic) is a modified form of the herpes virus made in a lab. T-VEC is a type of viral immunotherapy that uses a genetically formed virus to stimulate the body's immune system. It is injected directly into a tumor. T-VEC destroys tumor cells and also helps your body find and attack nearby cancer cells. Some side effects of T-VEC include fever, headaches, chills, muscle aches, and feeling tired and weak. Most people — about 9 out of 10 — who receive T-VEC develop flu-like symptoms, which usually get better after a few days.

TIL

Tumor-infiltrating lymphocyte (TIL) therapy (Lifileucel, Amtagvi) is an immune cell treatment that is approved as a second-line therapy. It uses the person's own cancer-fighting T cells, called tumor-infiltrating lymphocytes. These cells are collected from a person's own tumor in a lab. Once isolated from the tumor sample, the TILs are grown into the billions and infused back into the person. TIL is used for melanoma that has progressed on prior immunotherapy and targeted therapy (if the melanoma has a *BRAF* mutation). It is a specialized type of cellular therapy that is given only in approved centers with experience in the technique.

Side effects are common and come from the chemotherapy that is given along with the TIL. They include anemia, high fever, and drops in levels of platelets and certain white blood cells. When used with IL-2, see side effects of IL-2. Most of the time, side effects resolve within a couple of weeks.

Chemotherapy

Chemotherapy kills fast-growing cells throughout the body, including both cancer cells and normal cells. Chemotherapy drugs are usually given through an injection into a vein (IV) or are taken as a pill (by mouth).

Because chemotherapy doesn't treat melanoma as well as immunotherapy and targeted therapy do, your care team will likely use those therapies first.

But if your disease does not respond to immunotherapy or targeted therapy, or if you have severe side effects, chemotherapy may be an option.

Chemotherapy drugs used to treat melanoma include:

- Carboplatin
- Cisplatin
- Dacarbazine (also called DTIC)
- Nab-paclitaxel
- Paclitaxel
- Temozolomide (Temodar)

Chemotherapy treatment may last several months. Side effects include tiredness, nausea or vomiting, loss of appetite, diarrhea, nerve damage, and hair loss. These side effects often go away after you finish treatment.

Read more about help for nausea and vomiting in *NCCN Guidelines for Patients: Nausea and Vomiting* at NCCN.org/patientguidelines and on the NCCN Patient Guides for Cancer app.

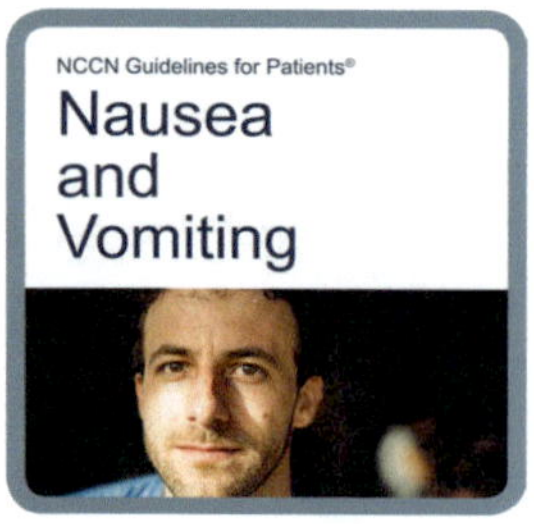

Radiation therapy

Radiation therapy focuses high-energy rays on tumor cells. The rays are delivered to the tumor area to damage the DNA inside the tumor cells. This either kills the tumor cells or stops new tumor cells from being made. You won't see, hear, or feel the radiation. It passes through your skin and other tissues to reach the tumor.

Radiation therapy can be given alone or with other treatments. Treatment may focus on individual tumors, a small area of the body, or a specific lymph node area. Radiation therapy can also be used as a palliative treatment to help ease pain or discomfort caused by cancer.

External beam radiation therapy (EBRT) is the most common method used. A large machine makes radiation beams that are directed at the tumor. The beams overlap at the site of the tumor or cancer cells to focus the high dose of radiation to that area. A much lower dose is given to nearby tissue. How often the treatment is given is based on the goal of your treatment and where the melanoma is located.

Intensity-modulated radiation therapy

Intensity-modulated radiation therapy (IMRT) uses many small beams of different strengths. This allows a high dose of radiation to be targeted at the tumor while limiting the amount of radiation to the surrounding normal tissue.

Image-guided radiation therapy

Image-guided RT (IGRT) uses imaging to deliver radiation to cancer. Imaging can confirm exactly where the tumor is in the body both before and during treatments.

Radiation therapy for distant disease

Other radiation techniques used to treat distant metastatic disease are:

Stereotactic radiosurgery (SRS) treats small tumors with very precise, high-dose x-ray beams and is usually finished in 1 session. It is preferred for brain metastases.

- Stereotactic radiotherapy (SRT) is a form of SRS and is finished in 1 to 5 sessions.
- SRT used to treat tumors in the body, and not in the brain, is sometimes called stereotactic body radiation therapy (SBRT) or stereotactic ablative body radiotherapy (SABR).

Side effects of radiation therapy may include:

- Sunburn-like skin problems
- Changes in skin color
- Hair loss around the area where radiation is given
- Fatigue
- Nausea if aimed at the abdomen (belly)

Clinical trials

Everyone with cancer should carefully consider all of the treatment options available for their cancer type, including standard treatments and clinical trials. Talk to your doctor about whether a clinical trial may make sense for you.

Phases

Most cancer clinical trials focus on treatment and are done in phases.

- **Phase 1 trials** study the safety and side effects of an investigational drug or treatment approach.
- **Phase 2 trials** study how well the drug or approach works against a specific type of cancer.
- **Phase 3 trials** test the drug or approach against a standard treatment. If the results are good, it may be approved by the FDA.
- **Phase 4 trials** study the safety and benefit of an FDA-approved treatment.

Who can enroll?

It depends on the clinical trial's rules, called eligibility criteria. The rules may be about age, cancer type and stage, treatment history, or general health. They ensure that participants are alike in specific ways and that the trial is as safe as possible for the participants.

Informed consent

Clinical trials are managed by a research team. This group of experts will review the study with you in detail, including its purpose and the risks and benefits of joining. All of this information is also provided in an informed consent form. Read the form carefully and ask questions before signing it. Take time to discuss it with people you trust. Keep in mind that you can leave and seek treatment outside of the clinical trial at any time.

Will I get a placebo?

Placebos (inactive versions of real medicines) are almost never used alone in cancer clinical trials. It is common to receive either a placebo with a standard treatment, or a new drug with a standard treatment. You will be informed, verbally and in writing, if a placebo is part of a clinical trial before you enroll.

Are clinical trials free?

There is no fee to enroll in a clinical trial. The study sponsor pays for research-related costs, including the study drug. But you may need to pay for other services, like transportation or childcare, due to extra appointments. During the trial, you will continue to receive standard cancer care. This care is often covered by insurance.

Finding a clinical trial

In the United States

NCCN Cancer Centers
NCCN.org/cancercenters

The National Cancer Institute (NCI)
cancer.gov/about-cancer/treatment/clinical-trials/search

Worldwide

The U.S. National Library of Medicine (NLM)
clinicaltrials.gov/

Need help finding a clinical trial?

NCI's Cancer Information Service (CIS)
1.800.4.CANCER (1.800.422.6237)
cancer.gov/contact

What's next

This chapter explained the types of treatments for melanoma. What treatment you receive will depend on the stage of melanoma. The next chapters are specific to the different stages of melanoma. At the end of the book, you'll see a *Follow-up care* chapter (Chapter 9) that describes how you'll be followed by your care team after treatment and how to prevent further skin cancers.

Key points

- Treatment for melanoma is based on the stage and location.
- Surgery is usually the primary (first) treatment for melanoma that has not spread.
- A wide excision surgery removes the melanoma tumor as well as some normal-looking tissue surrounding it.
- A sentinel lymph node biopsy (SLNB) removes nodes that are the most likely to have cancer if the cancer has spread. They will be checked for cancer cells by a pathologist.
- A lymph node dissection (removal) may be done if nearby lymph nodes are larger than normal.
- Targeted therapy drugs target the activity of a specific or unique feature of melanoma cancer cells.
- Immunotherapy improves your body's ability to find and destroy cancer cells. It can be given on its own or in combination with other types of treatment.

Questions to ask

- How will I be involved in making decisions for my treatment?
- Should I bring someone with me to the appointments?
- Can you explain the treatment and side effects as simply as possible?

5

Treatment for stages 0 to 2: Early stage

This chapter explains the early stages of melanoma — when most melanomas are diagnosed. It provides an overview of the best course of treatment and follow-up care.

In situ means "in place" in Latin. With melanoma, it means the cancer hasn't spread.

The early stages of melanoma (stages 0 through stage 2) is when the cancer is highly treatable and curable. After your biopsy confirms melanoma and its stage, you will need a physical exam and medical history with your provider. You will only need imaging tests if you have any unusual symptoms or if it might help with planning for surgery or systemic therapy. Keep reading to find out more about how the melanoma's stage reflects what treatment you may receive.

Stage 0 in situ

Stage 0 in situ refers to melanoma that is found only in the top layer of skin (epidermis). The melanoma at this stage is very unlikely to spread to other parts of the body. It is cured when completely removed.

Treatment

The standard treatment for stage 0 in situ is wide excision surgery. Wide excision surgery removes the melanoma tumor as well as some normal-looking tissue surrounding it (the surgical margin).

There are some areas where it is harder to do surgery, such as on the face, ears, palms of the hands, and soles of the feet. In these cases, your doctor might consider alternative surgical techniques, like Mohs micrographic surgery (or Mohs surgery). This type of surgery can provide a closer look at the edge of the removed tissue (called the histologic margin). With Mohs surgery, the surgeon removes thin layers of skin — one at a time — and checks each layer for cancer until reaching a layer where all the cancer cells are gone.

Additional treatment options for certain types of melanoma in situ (specifically the lentigo maligna type) include a topical immunotherapy cream called imiquimod. This topical treatment may be used if surgery isn't an option or if it fails to remove the tumor. While not commonly used, radiation therapy is another option for in situ melanoma.

Guide 5 Possible treatment for early-stage melanoma
Wide excision surgery
Wide excision surgery with SLNB
Immunotherapy
Radiation therapy
Clinical trials

Follow-up
Recommended steps after treatment for stage 0 melanoma include a medical history and skin exams at least once a year, which may help detect other skin cancers. You won't need imaging tests and blood tests.

Stage 1

Stage 1 melanoma has moved into the second layer of skin called the dermis. When melanoma reaches the dermis, it is described as invasive. Stage 1 is defined as a lesion (tumor) that is thinner than or equal to 2 mm (Breslow depth or thickness). Stage 1 melanoma may or may not be ulcerated (broken skin), though most are not. Stage 1 melanoma has two subgroups: 1A and 1B.

Stage 1A

This stage is defined as a tumor that is less than 0.8 mm thick and doesn't have a break on the skin (ulceration) when examined under the microscope. It is considered still localized to the skin, but is invasive, which means that it has gone through the top layer of skin into the next layer of skin.

Treatment
Wide excision surgery is used to treat stage 1A melanoma. Sentinel lymph node biopsy (SLNB) is usually not recommended at this stage.

Follow-up
Recommended steps after treatment for stage 1A melanoma include a physical exam and medical history, with a focus on the skin and regional lymph nodes near the primary melanoma site, every 6 to 12 months for 5 years, and then at least once every year afterward. Imaging tests will be done only to check for specific signs and symptoms.

Stage 1B

In stage 1B melanoma, the primary tumor has moved into the lower layer of skin but is still curable. Stage 1B includes tumors that are:

Early stage melanoma is highly treatable. Be sure to ask questions if you need more information.

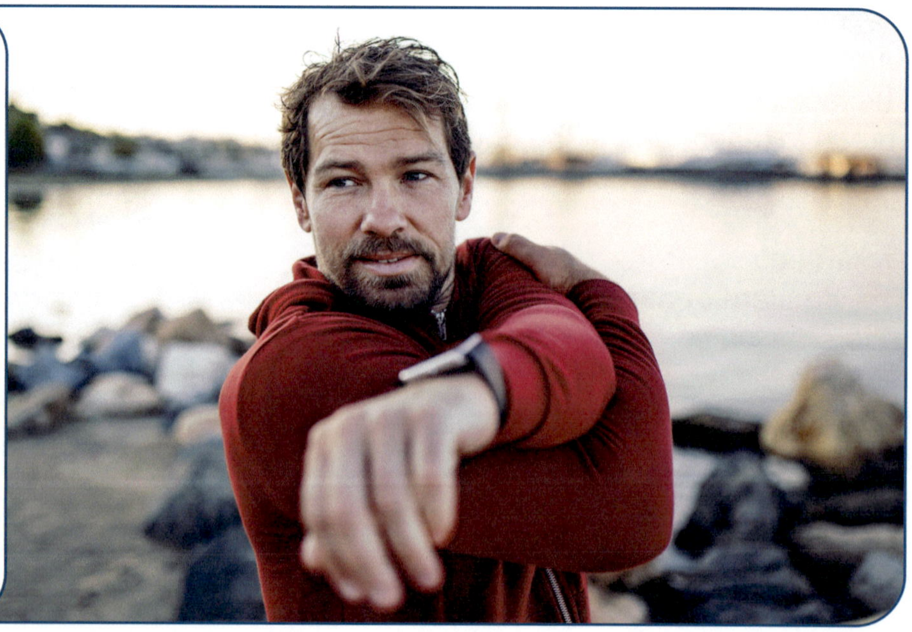

- Less than 0.8 mm thick with ulceration
- Between 0.8 and 1 mm thick with or without ulceration
- Between 1 and 2 mm thick without ulceration

Keep reading for treatment as stage 1B is treated mostly the same as stage 2A.

Stage 2

Stage 2 refers to tumors that are 1 to 2 mm in thickness and are ulcerated, or tumors that are thicker than 2 mm with or without ulceration. A person with stage 2 melanoma has a higher chance of cancer spreading beyond the primary tumor than a person with stage 1 melanoma.

Stage 2 melanoma is broken down into three subgroups: 2A, 2B, and 2C.

Stage 2A

Stage 2A melanoma includes two types of tumors:

- Between 1 and 2 mm thick with ulceration
- Between 2 and 4 mm thick without ulceration

Treatment

Primary treatment for stage 1B through stage 2A is mostly the same and includes wide excision surgery. Your provider may discuss performing an SLNB along with wide excision surgery. See *Chapter 4: Treatment overview* for more information on SLNB.

If your provider doesn't think the melanoma requires an SLNB, then you will have standard wide excision surgery. After that, you will be observed on a regular schedule (see *Follow-up*).

Whether or not your provider thinks you should have an SLNB, the decision will be made with you. It will be based on any health conditions you have, your age and general health, and your personal preferences. If the melanoma meets the criteria for SLNB, the procedure will find out whether cancer cells are in one or more nearby lymph nodes (**see Guide 6**).

Your provider may consider nodal basin ultrasound imaging before the SLNB, if results of the physical exam were unclear. Even if the nodal basin ultrasound doesn't indicate cancer in the nodes, you may still need an SLNB. Other imaging might also be ordered if you have signs or symptoms of cancer.

If you have a negative result from the SLNB, it means the cancer has not spread to nearby lymph nodes. If the melanoma is stage 1B or 2A and no cancer is found in lymph nodes, you may start follow-up care (see *Follow-up*) as no further treatment is generally needed.

However, a positive SLNB result shows that cancer is present in the sentinel lymph nodes and that other lymph nodes may be affected.

If the SLNB finds cancer in lymph nodes, the cancer stage will be changed (upstaged) to stage 3. The cancer will also be upstaged to stage 3 if very tiny tumors, called microscopic satellites, are found in the surgical margin. For more information on stage 3 melanoma treatment, see *Chapter 6: Treatment for stage 3: Regional.*

Follow-up

Recommended steps after treatment for stage 1B to 2A melanoma include physical exams and medical history with a focus on the skin and regional lymph nodes, every 6 to 12 months for 5 years, and then every year afterward as needed. Imaging tests will be done only to evaluate specific signs and symptoms to see if the cancer has recurred (returned).

Stage 2B or stage 2C

Stage 2B melanoma is defined as a lesion (tumor) that is thicker than 2 mm but no thicker than 4 mm with ulceration, or the melanoma is thicker than 4 mm without ulceration.

Stage 2C means the melanoma is thicker than 4 mm, and the outermost layer of skin covering the tumor is ulcerated.

Treatment

Primary treatment for stage 2B or 2C is the same and involves wide excision surgery and SLNB. Imaging with PET/CT or CT of

Guide 6
When you might have a sentinel lymph node biopsy (SLNB)

A sentinel lymph node is the first lymph node where cancer cells spread after leaving a tumor. An SLNB shows if cancer has spread from a tumor. It helps providers tell the stage of the melanoma and can help you and your care team make treatment decisions.

You might need an SLNB if:

Your cancer is stage 1A and:	• The melanoma is less than 0.8 mm deep • The melanoma has no breakage (ulceration) or other features	**Your doctor will not likely recommend an SLNB.**
Your cancer is stage 1B and:	• The melanoma is less than 0.8 mm deep and has ulceration • The melanoma is 0.8 to 1 mm deep with or without ulceration	**Your doctor might recommend an SLNB.**
Your cancer is stage 1B or higher and:	• The melanoma is more than 1 mm deep • You had an in-transit metastasis or local recurrence of a melanoma but no sign of regional or distant metastases	**Your doctor will likely recommend an SLNB.**

the chest, abdomen, and pelvis may be done beforehand if it's needed to plan surgery. You might need imaging if you have any unusual signs or symptoms that need further work up. Imaging can also help guide shared decision making between you and your medical oncologist regarding adjuvant systemic therapy after surgery. An SLNB is typically recommended for complete (pathological) staging and is strongly recommended before adjuvant immunotherapy with pembrolizumab or nivolumab.

Following surgery and if no cancer is found in sentinel lymph nodes, close follow-up care is recommended and may include imaging scans to help detect melanoma recurrence. After talking with a medical oncologist, some people choose to receive adjuvant therapy with pembrolizumab or nivolumab. (Though not used often, you may receive radiation therapy to areas where tumors are likely to return.)

Adjuvant pembrolizumab or nivolumab can help reduce the chance of cancer returning. However, you could experience long-term immunotherapy-related side effects.

Your doctor should discuss with you the pros and cons of pembrolizumab or nivolumab for treatment. Factors to consider, in addition to the stage of the disease, include your age, how active you are, your personal and family history of autoimmune disease, and how toxic systemic therapies might be for you.

If cancer is found in the SLNB, the melanoma will be upstaged to stage 3. For more information on stage 3 treatment options, see *Chapter 6: Treatment for stage 3: Regional*.

"Knowing there is treatment available gave me hope at diagnosis and for the future."

Follow-up

Recommended steps after treatment for stage 2B and 2C melanomas include a physical exam and medical history, with a focus on the skin and lymph nodes. Follow-up visits should occur every 3 to 6 months for 2 years, and then every 3 to 12 months for 3 years, then yearly after that point.

Imaging tests will be done to evaluate any concerning signs and symptoms, and usually after receiving adjuvant treatment. Your doctor may consider imaging tests every 3 to 12 months for 2 years, and then every 6 to 12 months for another 1 to 3 years to look for the recurrence (return) or metastasis (spread) of melanoma.

What's next

This chapter explained treatments for early-stage melanoma. At these stages, melanoma is often curable. After successful treatment, regular follow-up care is needed. Be sure to check out the last chapter (Chapter 9) to learn more about follow-up care, your genetic risk and genetic testing, and preventing skin cancer.

Key points

- Stage 0 through stage 2 melanomas are considered early-stage cancer. They are highly treatable and curable.
- The standard treatment for stage 0 in situ and stage 1A melanoma is wide excision surgery.
- A sentinel lymph node biopsy (SLNB) may be done in addition to wide excision surgery for stage 1B and stage 2 melanoma.
- If cancer is found in the SLNB, you will be upstaged to stage 3 melanoma.
- Adjuvant therapy (after primary treatment) may be used for stage 2 melanoma. It can help reduce the chance of cancer returning.
- If you are considered for adjuvant therapy, pretreatment imaging may be needed to help guide treatment.
- Depending on your signs and symptoms after treatment, you may undergo monitoring of your skin and lymph nodes for up to 3 years.

Questions to ask

- What are the chances of the melanoma coming back after my treatment?
- Will insurance cover my treatment?
- Should I be using a patient portal to get my test results?
- How long until I receive test results after an SLNB?

6

Treatment for stage 3: Regional

Stage 3 melanoma is considered an advanced form of cancer. In this stage, the melanoma has spread to the nearby lymph nodes, lymph vessels, or other parts of the skin but has not spread further than that. There are many treatment options depending on the features of the melanoma.

Stage 3

Stage 3 melanoma means the cancer has spread from the main skin tumor to nearby areas. It is called regional melanoma because the cancer has spread locally but not to distant parts of the body. Stage 3 melanoma has 1 or more of these 4 features:

- **Nearby lymph nodes with cancer** may be found. Lymph nodes are small bean-shaped structures that help fight disease. (When distant nodes have cancer, the cancer is stage 4.)
- **Microscopic satellites (microsatellites)** are tiny skin tumors that are next to or below the main skin tumor and can be seen only with a microscope.
- **Satellite tumors** are deposits of melanoma in the lymph vessels no more than 2 cm from the main tumor. They are large enough to be seen or felt during a skin exam.
- **In-transit tumors** are lymph vessel deposits that are farther than 2 cm from the main tumor but haven't reached the lymph nodes.

For more information, see *Chapter 3: Staging for melanoma.*

Features and subgroups

Stage 3 cancer is further broken down into 4 subgroups: 3A, 3B, 3C, and 3D. Each subgroup describes the extent of stage 3 melanoma. Stage 3A is less advanced melanoma while stage 3D is more advanced.

The way stage 3 is treated depends on its features, which help determine the subgroup.

Stage 3A

Stage 3A melanoma includes the tumors that may be:

- 1 mm thick or less with or without ulceration (broken skin)
- 2 mm thick or less without ulceration

This stage also means that between 1 to 3 lymph nodes have cancer detected microscopically after a sentinel lymph node biopsy (SLNB).

Stage 3B

Stage 3B indicates tumors that have:

- Thickness that can be less than 1 mm or up to 4 mm with or without ulceration;
- 1 to 3 lymph nodes found by physical exam or imaging tests

- Microsatellite tumors, satellite tumors, or in-transit metastases on or under the skin.

Stage 3C

A stage 3C tumor is identified as:

- Less than 2 mm thick to more than 4 mm thick with or without ulceration
- Involving anywhere from 1 to 4 lymph nodes found by physical exam or imaging tests; and/or any number of lymph nodes clumped together
- Having microsatellite tumors, satellite tumors, or in-transit metastases on or under the skin

Stage 3D

Stage 3D indicates the tumor is:

- More than 4 mm thick with ulceration
- Found with cancer in 4 or more lymph nodes or any number of lymph nodes clumped (matted) together
- Associated with 2 or more lymph nodes and/or any number of lymph nodes clumped together. There are also microsatellite tumors, satellite tumors, and/or in-transit metastases on or under the skin

Ask your care team to explain why the melanoma is stage 3. You may also be able to find this information in pathology reports.

All follow-up care is the same for stage 3 and mentioned at the end of this chapter.

Satellite and in-transit tumors

Melanoma cells can spread from the main tumor through the lymph system. This system consists of small vessels and bean-shaped structures called lymph nodes (shown in green). Melanoma may form one or more satellite tumors, which are close to the main tumor. In-transit tumors are farther away but haven't reached nearby lymph nodes.

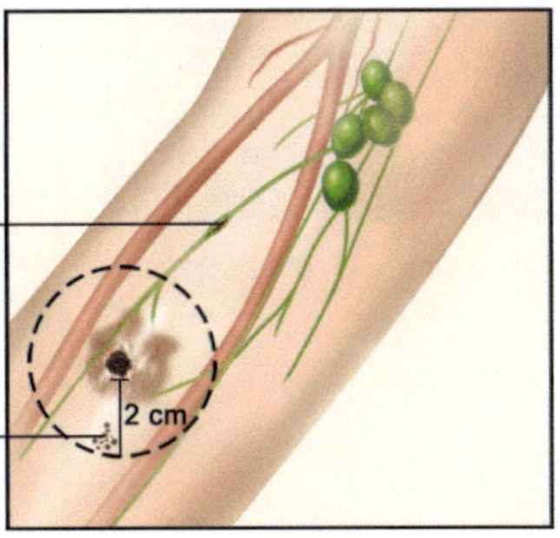

Microsatellite tumors (only seen with a microscope)

Cancer in nearby lymph nodes is a common feature of stage 3 melanoma. There are two ways that cancer is found in the lymph nodes:

- The pathologist confirmed cancer in abnormal nodes that were detected by a physical exam or imaging and biopsied before treatment
- The pathologist found cancer in the SLNB

Cancer in the sentinel nodes

A sentinel lymph node is the first lymph node where cancer cells most likely spread from a primary tumor. When cancer is found in sentinel lymph nodes, it is called sentinel node positive. Testing and treatment depends on the number of nodes with cancer.

Tests

For stage 3A, your care team may consider imaging to help with staging. For stages 3B, 3C, or 3D that have cancer in sentinel nodes, imaging for staging is recommended. If melanoma involves the lymph nodes or other parts of the body, *BRAF* V600 mutation testing is considered to determine whether targeted therapy is an option.

When sentinel lymph nodes have cancer, other nearby nodes may have cancer, too. Cancer care options include a series of imaging tests to check nearby lymph nodes called the nodal basin.

Treatment

Active nodal basin ultrasound or other types of imaging (CT, PET-CT, or MRI) without further lymph node removal (called complete lymph node dissection or CLND) are considered the preferred treatment for cancer in the sentinel nodes. **See Guide 7**. CLND should only be used for certain people and circumstances because of its risk of severe side effects like lymphedema (swelling due to buildup of lymph fluid in the fatty tissue just under your skin near the surgery site). CLND also involves extensive surgery, longer recovery time, and hospitalization. If signs of cancer appear, adjuvant (after surgery) treatment can be received at that time.

For most 3A tumors, no further treatment is required. Instead, observation is the preferred next treatment. Observation means periodic doctor visits that include skin and lymph node exams, attention to any concerning signs and symptoms, and/or imaging scans, when needed.

But the next step for cancer in the sentinel nodes, especially for Stage 3B, 3C or 3D, could be adjuvant treatment. Before choosing one of the adjuvant systemic therapies, your care team should consider both your risk of cancer recurrence (returning) and how toxic the systemic therapies might be for you.

Guide 7 Possible treatment for cancer in sentinel nodes
Active nodal basin ultrasound without CLND
CLND (for select patients)
Systemic therapy
Observation

If the cancer is considered low risk, for example, the toxicity of adjuvant therapy may outweigh any potential benefit you might receive from the treatment. Because of that, adjuvant therapy may not be recommended.

But if your doctor recommends adjuvant therapy, options are:

- Nivolumab
- Pembrolizumab
- Dabrafenib/trametinib or other BRAF or MEK inhibitors for people with *BRAF* V600 mutation

As mentioned previously, another option is undergoing observation in the follow-up phase.

After all treatment, you will move to follow-up care. See *Follow-up for stage 3.*

Cancer in the lymph nodes

Your care team may have detected abnormal lymph nodes before you started treatment, possibly during your physical exam or through imaging. Then a biopsy, either needle (preferred) or excisional (called complete), confirmed cancer in these nodes, which are referred to as clinically positive lymph nodes. Melanoma at this stage could be 3B, 3C, or 3D.

Tests

Further recommended tests to guide treatment are:

- Imaging for staging and to assess signs or symptoms of cancer
- *BRAF* V600 mutation testing

Your care team will discuss and decide if surgery can remove all the melanoma

Guide 8
Treatment of melanoma with clinically positive nodes

If cancer can be treated with surgery (resectable)	Treatment may include three phases: • Neoadjuvant therapy with immunotherapy, targeted therapy, or both • Surgery with a wide excision and therapeutic lymph node dissection (TLND) • Adjuvant therapy with systemic drugs, radiation therapy, or observation
If cancer can't be treated with surgery (unresectable)	• Systemic therapy is the preferred option • Radiation therapy (palliative) for symptom relief • T-VEC skin injection • Best supportive care

(meaning it's resectable). **See Guide 8** for treatment options.

Treatment

Before surgery, you may receive drug treatment to improve outcomes. This treatment is called neoadjuvant therapy. Neoadjuvant therapy may consist of immunotherapy, targeted therapy, or both.

Clinical trials have shown a benefit to receiving neoadjuvant therapy before surgery. But experts are still studying which drugs work best, in which people, and how long treatment is needed.

- Preferred therapies have the most evidence they work better and may be safer than other therapies. Preferred drug options for neoadjuvant therapy include pembrolizumab, or nivolumab and ipilimumab. (Only IV nivolumab can be used with ipilimumab, not the injectable form.)
- Other recommended therapies may not work quite as well as preferred therapies, but they can still help treat cancer. Other recommended options for neoadjuvant therapy include nivolumab with or without relatlimab.
- Therapies used in certain cases work best for people with specific cancer features or health circumstances. One such neoadjuvant treatment is dabrafenib or trametinib for people who have *BRAF* V600 mutation.

Important to know: Sometimes other targeted therapy combinations can be considered if the side effects are too much for you (known as toxicity).

Another treatment option is to have surgery, which consists of a wide excision of the tumor while removing nearby lymph nodes. This is called a therapeutic lymph node dissection (TLND). The number of lymph nodes removed depends on the involved lymph node basin.

TLND is recommended if you had neoadjuvant therapy first or it can be done without neoadjuvant therapy if neoadjuvant therapy isn't an option for you.

After surgery, your care team will decide if more treatment may help stop the cancer from returning. Treatment after surgery is called adjuvant therapy.

If the cancer is likely to return, the preferred adjuvant systemic therapy options include:

- Nivolumab
- Pembrolizumab

Systemic therapy travels in your bloodstream to treat cancer anywhere in the body.

Adjuvant therapy is sometimes used in addition to primary treatments to boost their effectiveness.

- Dabrafenib/trametinib (if you have *BRAF* V600 mutation)

You may also receive adjuvant radiation therapy, although its use has mostly been replaced by the cancer drugs listed above. Adjuvant radiation therapy is not often recommended since it only treats the region where the lymph nodes were removed and not other areas.

One other option is observation and is based on your care team's decision of the risk of the melanoma's recurrence and the risk of treatment side effects (toxicity).

Observation involves periodic doctor visits that include skin and lymph node exams, attention to any concerning signs and symptoms, and/or imaging scans, when needed.

But if surgery is not an option (and the tumor is considered unresectable), the preferred treatment is systemic therapy (**see Guide 16**, *Chapter 8: Treatment for stage 4: Metastatic disease,* for therapies).

In addition, you may get relief from one or more of these treatments:

- Palliative radiation therapy
- T-VEC (virus that is injected into the skin tumor and triggers your body to find and attack nearby cancer cells)
- Best supportive care, also known as palliative care

Microsatellites

Stage 3 melanoma may involve microscopic satellites (microsatellites) so named because these tiny tumors can only be seen with a microscope. Stage 3A does not involve microsatellites. But if microsatellites are found in the biopsy of a 3A melanoma, it can be upstaged as a pathological stage 3B melanoma. For all stages, microsatellites are found in either:

- A skin biopsy sample removed before treatment
- The tissue removed during surgery

Tests

The tests for melanoma with microscopic satellites include:

- Imaging tests for staging
- Imaging tests to assess signs or symptoms of cancer

Guide 9 Possible treatment for cancer with microsatellites
Wide excision surgery
Wide excision with SLNB
Clinical trial
Observation
Systemic therapy

- *BRAF* mutation testing if you might have adjuvant therapy (described below) or enroll in a clinical trial

Once tests have been completed, your doctor may discuss having a sentinel lymph node biopsy (SLNB) to see if the cancer has spread to the lymph nodes. An SLNB will remove the tissue from the first lymph nodes where fluid from the tumor drains.

Treatment

Primary treatment will be wide excision surgery and possibly an SLNB. If you had a wide excision before, your care team may think it's best to forego an SLNB, which is ideally done at the same time as the wide excision. **See Guide 9.**

After surgery, you may have more treatment called adjuvant therapy. Adjuvant therapy treats any cancer cells that may have been left behind. If you didn't have an SLNB or you had one and no cancer was found in lymph nodes, options include participation in a clinical trial or systemic therapy with:

- Nivolumab
- Pembrolizumab
- Dabrafenib and trametinib (but only if you have *BRAF* V600 mutation)

Observation is also an option. Observation involves having regular doctor visits that include skin and lymph node exams, attention to any concerning signs and symptoms, and/or imaging scans, when needed.

Satellite or in-transit tumors

Melanoma may spread and form nearby skin tumors called satellite or in-transit tumors. These tumors are seen or felt during the skin exam and then confirmed by biopsy to be cancer.

Tests

Other recommended tests to determine if surgery is necessary include:

- Imaging for staging and to assess signs or symptoms of cancer
- *BRAF* mutation testing if not already done

When the cancer can be removed with surgery, it is called resectable. Cancer that cannot be treated with surgery is called unresectable. Sometimes satellite/in-transit tumors can be considered either resectable or unresectable/borderline resectable. Unresectable/borderline resectable means the tumor is on the border (outside limit) of what surgery might be able to accomplish. Resectable means the tumor

Guide 10 Possible treatment for cancer with satellite or in-transit tumors
Neoadjuvant systemic therapy
Surgery (complete excision) to clear margins
T-VEC/intralesional therapy
Systemic therapy
Radiation therapy
Observation

could be surgically removed if treatment shrinks the tumor first.

Treatment: Resectable disease

There are four options in initial treatment for resectable cancer:

- Neoadjuvant systemic therapy (**see Guide 11**)
- Surgery (complete excision) to clear margins
- T-VEC/intralesional therapy
- Systemic therapy (**see Guide 16**, *Chapter 8: Treatment for stage 4: Metastatic disease,* for options)

Surgery with neoadjuvant therapy

If you received neoadjuvant systemic therapy to shrink the tumor, the next step is surgery. The cancer will be removed with complete excision to clear margins. Clear margins means there is no evidence (signs) of disease (cancer) on the edges of the surgical excision as well as elsewhere.

Following surgery, the preferred options for adjuvant systemic therapy include: nivolumab, pembrolizumab, or dabrafenib and trametinib if you have *BRAF* V600 mutation.

One other option is observation. This involves regular clinical exams and imaging scans for any new cancer signs or symptoms.

Surgery without neoadjuvant therapy

If you received a complete excision to clear margins as initial treatment without neoadjuvant systemic therapy and there are no signs of remaining cancer cells, you might receive the adjuvant systemic treatment options or observation.

If cancer cells remain after complete excision, read the section ahead on unresectable/borderline resectable disease for treatment options.

Guide 11
Neoadjuvant (before surgery) systemic therapy options

Preferred options	• Pembrolizumab • Nivolumab/ipilimumab*
Other recommended options	• Nivolumab • Nivolumab and relatlimab
Used in some cases	• Dabrafenib/trametinib if *BRAF* V600 mutation positive

*only IV nivolumab can be used with ipilimumab, not the injectable form

Systemic therapy and T-VEC

If you receive systemic therapy or T-VEC/intralesional therapy as your initial treatment, you may receive any combination of clinical exams (skin exam or physical exam), a pathologic assessment (like another biopsy) or imaging to determine the cancer's response to the treatment.

If there is still cancer present that is considered unresectable and progressive after those therapies, then you will be treated following the unresectable/borderline resectable disease treatment in the next section.

But if there is cancer remaining that is resectable, you will likely have the same treatment (one of the four options) for resectable disease, noted above, or possibly another treatment like radiation.

No evidence of disease after T-VEC

If there is no evidence of disease after T-VEC/intralesional therapy and further exams, then your provider will likely consider one of these adjuvant therapy options:

- Nivolumab
- Pembrolizumab
- Dabrafenib/trametinib if you have *BRAF* V600 mutation
- Observation

If there's no evidence of disease after you've had systemic therapy as an initial treatment and further exams, you will move to observation as part of follow-up.

Treatment: Unresectable/borderline resectable disease

Instead of upfront surgery because it's considered unresectable/borderline resectable, initial treatment options include systemic therapy, which is preferred (**see Guide 16**, *Chapter 8: Treatment for stage 4: Metastatic disease*).

Or you could have local therapy options such as:

- Intralesional injection options:
  - T-VEC, which is preferred
  - Interleukin-2 (IL-2), which is a type of injectable immunotherapy and only helpful in some cases
- Radiation therapy might be considered
- Palliative (limited) surgery or local ablation (minimally invasive) therapy

Regional chemotherapy is another option for local satellite/in-transit melanoma that's confined to an arm or leg. The treatment is called isolated limb infusion or isolated limb perfusion (ILI/ILP) with melphalan and treats just the limb involved with the melanoma. This procedure should only be done at centers experienced in providing ILI/ILP.

After treatment, your doctor may perform another skin exam or biopsy and you may undergo imaging. The next treatment is based on those test results:

- If some cancer remains and appears to be unresectable, you may have the same treatment as in the initial treatment section.

- If there is some resectable melanoma remaining, you will have the same treatment as resectable disease.
- If there are no signs of cancer after local or regional therapy, you may start adjuvant systemic therapy (nivolumab, pembrolizumab or dabrafenib/trametinib if you have *BRAF* V600 mutation) or start observation with periodic imaging.
- If no cancer remains after systemic therapy, you will move to observation as part of follow-up care.

Follow-up for stage 3

For all stage 3 melanoma, follow-up care involves ongoing testing for new signs and symptoms of cancer, also known as observation. It is described in *Chapter 9: Follow-up care*. Follow up starts when there are no signs of cancer after treatment.

Supportive Care

Supportive care helps improve your quality of life during and after cancer treatment. The goal is to prevent or manage side effects and symptoms, like pain and cancer-related fatigue. It also addresses the mental, social, and spiritual concerns faced by those with cancer.

Supportive care is available to everyone with cancer and their families, not just those at the end of life. Palliative care is another name for supportive care.

Supportive care can also help with:

- Making treatment decisions
- Coordinating your care
- Paying for care
- Planning for advanced care and end of life

If you need support while dealing with a melanoma diagnosis, find a nearby in-person or online cancer support group.

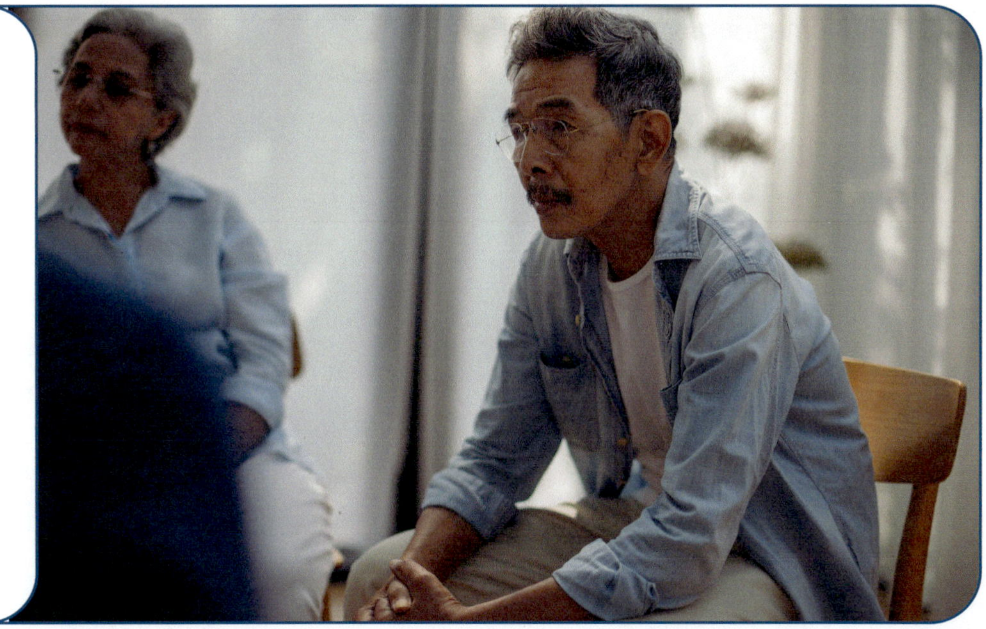

Recommended follow-up tests for stage 3 melanoma include:

- Physical exam and medical history with a focus on the skin and lymph nodes, every 3 to 6 months for 2 years, then every 3 to 12 months for 3 years, and then every year as needed.
- Imaging tests as needed based on cancer signs and symptoms. Imaging might occur every 3 to 12 months for 2 years, then every 6 to 12 months for another 3 years.
- After 3 to 5 years, routine imaging is not recommended.

What's next

In this chapter, you learned about stage 3 melanoma, which is considered regional. It has spread locally and not far in the body. The next step is regular follow-up care to prevent and find another skin cancer. Read *Chapter 9: Follow-up care* for more information on what that might look like and about how you can spot and prevent skin cancers, as well as information about genetic risks. If the melanoma returns, it's called recurrence. For more information on if the melanoma comes back, read the next chapter *(Chapter 7: Treatment for recurrence)*.

Key points

- Stage 3 melanoma has spread to nearby lymph nodes, lymph vessels, or skin areas.
- Tests for stage 3 melanoma include imaging and often *BRAF* mutation testing.
- Microscopic satellites are tiny tumors that can only be seen with a microscope.
- When cancer is found in sentinel lymph nodes, signs of cancer in other nodes may be assessed with ultrasound or other imaging, or more nodes may be removed.
- Melanoma that is found in enlarged lymph nodes can often be treated with surgery.
- Neoadjuvant therapy is often recommended to shrink a tumor prior to surgery and then can be followed by adjuvant therapy.
- Melanoma may spread and form more skin tumors called satellite or in-transit tumors.

Questions to ask

- How far has the cancer spread?
- Will I need genetic testing?
- What are the side effects from systemic therapies?
- Should I bring someone with me to appointments?

7 Treatment for recurrence

When cancer comes back after treatment, it's called recurrent cancer. This chapter reviews the different types of melanoma recurrence, as well as testing and treatment options.

When melanoma recurs, it often doesn't look like the original melanoma. Many times, the melanoma appears as lumps under the skin or in the lymph nodes. Early-stage melanoma is less likely to recur than advanced melanoma. Most recurrences happen within 3 years after treatment. If the recurrence is a distant metastasis, read *Chapter 8: Treatment for stage 4: Metastatic disease* for options.

True scar recurrence

True scar recurrence, also known as persistent disease, is a tumor next to the scar tissue from the melanoma surgery. It occurs because not all of the melanoma was removed during surgery despite best efforts.

This tumor looks like the original melanoma. It is often found in the top layers of the skin (epidermis or superficial dermis).

Tests

Testing for true scar recurrence includes a skin biopsy to confirm it's cancer. The next tests you will receive are based on the stage and features of the recurrent melanoma. Tests could include lymphatic mapping (the use of dyes and radioactive substances to identify cancer in lymph nodes) or sentinel lymph node biopsy (SLNB). Ask your care team about any additional testing you may have.

Treatment

Treatment options for true scar recurrence include:

- Surgery to remove the tumor, with surgical margins based on the tumor depth (Breslow thickness)
- SLNB based on lymphatic mapping if the tumor grew near lymph vessels

Depending on how advanced the recurrence is, your care team might also recommend:

- Clinical trial (for stage 2, if available)
- Observation with or without surveillance imaging
- Pembrolizumab or nivolumab for pathologically staged 2B or 2C
- Primary tumor site radiation therapy

Guide 12 Possible treatment for true scar recurrence
Re-excision of tumor site
Lymphatic mapping or SLNB
Radiation therapy
Immunotherapy
Observation

Local satellite and in-transit recurrence

Local satellite recurrence and in-transit recurrence both mean the cancer has returned in the lymph vessels. It is usually found either within or surrounding the primary melanoma scar. Local satellite recurrence can feel like a firm bump in or around that area.

In-transit recurrence is usually found between the primary site and regional lymph nodes. It means the cancer has returned and formed tumors in the lymph vessels between the melanoma scar site and the regional lymph nodes, but not in the lymph nodes themselves.

These two types of recurrence are tested and treated the same way.

Tests

Testing for local satellite or in-transit recurrence includes these options:

- Core biopsy (the preferred option) or fine-needle aspiration, incisional (partial) biopsy, or excisional (complete) biopsy
- Imaging to assess cancer signs or symptoms
- *BRAF* mutation testing, if not already done

Treatment of recurrent satellite or in-transit tumors is almost the same as the treatment for these tumors when found at diagnosis. (For treatment at diagnosis, see *Chapter 6: Treatment for stage 3: Regional.*) Treatment of recurrence depends on if the cancer can be removed with surgery (resectable disease) or not (unresectable/borderline resectable).

Treatment: Resectable

When the recurrent cancer has resectable disease, your first treatment options may be:

- Neoadjuvant systemic therapy (**see Guide 11**)
- Surgery with complete excision to clear margins and removal of all disease
- T-VEC/intralesional therapy
- Systemic therapy (**see Guide 16** in *Chapter 8: Treatment for stage 4: Metastatic disease*)

After surgery to clear margins and there is no evidence of disease, you could have one of the preferred adjuvant therapy options:

- Nivolumab
- Pembrolizumab

Guide 13 Possible treatment for local satellite and in-transit recurrence
Neoadjuvant systemic therapy
Surgery (complete excision) to clear margins
T-VEC/intralesional therapy
Systemic therapy
Adjuvant systemic therapy
Regional therapy
Palliation (limited excision or local ablation)
Observation

- Dabrafenib/trametinib if you have *BRAF* V600 mutation
- If you had anti-PD-1 therapy, you might have ipilimumab

If the surgery is not able to completely remove the cancer, you will follow the treatment in the unresectable/borderline resectable section.

But if you received T-VEC or systemic therapy as initial treatment, your provider may recommend another biopsy and more imaging to see if your cancer is responding to treatment.

At that point, if there is residual/progressive unresectable disease, you will receive the same treatment as unresectable/borderline resectable section.

But if there is residual disease that is resectable, then you might receive one of four treatment options:

- Neoadjuvant systemic therapy (**see Guide 11**, Chapter 6)
- Complete excision to clear margins
- T-VEC/intralesional therapy
- Systemic therapy (**see Guide 16**, Chapter 8)

Still, if you've had local or regional therapy and the cancer shows no evidence of disease, then you could have one of the preferred adjuvant therapy options:

- Nivolumab
- Pembrolizumab
- Dabrafenib/trametinib if you have *BRAF* V600 mutation

Neoadjuvant therapy is used to reduce cancer before the main treatment.

- Ipilimumab (if you had anti-PD-1 therapy)

If no cancer remains after systemic therapy, you can begin follow-up care.

Treatment: Unresectable/ borderline resectable

When the melanoma can't be treated with surgery, it is unresectable/borderline resectable disease, and there are many other options. The preferred initial treatment is systemic therapy as described in *Chapter 8: Treatment for stage 4: Metastatic disease* (**see Guide 16**) for metastatic cancer.

Other treatment includes local therapy options, such as:

- Intralesional injection options (T-VEC, preferred)
- IL-2, used in some cases
- Radiation therapy
- Symptom relief (palliation), which can include limited excision or local ablation therapy

Regional therapy, such as isolated limb infusion/perfusion (ILI/ILP) with melphalan-based regimens, is another option for unresectable/borderline resectable recurrent disease. This is a procedure where a high dose of drugs is injected directly into a tumor in an arm or a leg and where the cancer is only in that limb. This therapy should only be done in centers with experience in ILI/ILP.

After initial treatment, your provider will examine you and may need to get more information in the form of another biopsy and more imaging to see if your cancer is responding to treatment.

The next treatment is based on those results:

- If some cancer remains and appears to be unresectable, you may have the same treatment as mentioned in the initial treatment section.
- If there is some resectable melanoma remaining, you will have the same treatment as the resectable disease, mentioned previously.
- If there are no signs of cancer after local or regional therapy, you may start adjuvant systemic therapy that could include:
    - Nivolumab
    - Pembrolizumab
    - Dabrafenib/trametinib if *BRAF* V600 mutation positive
    - Ipilimumab (if you had anti-PD-1 therapy)

If no cancer remains after systemic therapy, you move to observation in follow-up care. See *Chapter 9: Follow-up care.*

Nodal recurrence

Nodal recurrence means the cancer has returned and is found in your lymph nodes. It often appears as enlarged lymph nodes in the lymph node basin close to where the melanoma was located.

Tests

Testing for nodal recurrence can include:

- Core biopsy or fine-needle aspiration are preferred to confirm the diagnosis
- Imaging to see how much the disease has spread and to check cancer signs or symptoms
- *BRAF* mutation testing (if not already done)

Results from these tests will determine if the cancer is limited to the lymph nodes or if it has spread farther, known as metastatic disease.

If tests find the melanoma has spread farther than nearby lymph nodes, see *Chapter 8:*

Guide 14 Possible treatment for nodal recurrence
Neoadjuvant systemic therapy
Surgery (excision of recurrence) with TLND
Surgery (excision recurrence) without TLND
Adjuvant systemic therapy
Locoregional therapy
Observation

Treatment for stage 4: Metastatic disease to learn what treatment options are available.

If you have disease limited to the lymph nodes, treatment depends on whether you had a previous lymph node dissection (removal).

No previous lymph node removal (resectable)

If you had no previous lymph node removal and the cancer is considered resectable, you might first have neoadjuvant systemic therapy (**see Guide 11**, Chapter 6) before surgery to help shrink the tumor and to reduce risk of recurrence.

After neoadjuvant therapy, you'll have surgery to remove the enlarged lymph nodes. Other lymph nodes that may have cancer will be removed, too. This is called a therapeutic lymph node dissection (TLND).

Or you might not have neoadjuvant therapy and instead just have the surgery and TLND to remove the cancer recurrence in the lymph nodes.

After the surgery, you may receive adjuvant therapy, such as:

- One of the following preferred treatments: Nivolumab, pembrolizumab, dabrafenib/ trametinib or other BRAF or MEK inhibitors for people with *BRAF* V600 mutation
- Ipilimumab if you already had anti-PD-1 therapy, used in some cases

Palliative options mean they're intended to ease the suffering from cancer symptoms.

You might also have one or both of the following:

- Locoregional radiation therapy to nodal basin if you have a higher risk of another recurrence
- Observation as part of follow-up care.

For more information on follow-up care, see *Chapter 9: Follow-up care.*

No previous lymph node removal (unresectable)

If you didn't have a lymph node removal before, and the cancer is considered unresectable, then you will follow the same treatment as if you had a lymph node dissection below, see *Unresectable disease*.

Previous lymph node removal (resectable)

If the recurrent disease is limited to lymph nodes and you've had a lymph node removal before, then treatment for your remaining melanoma depends on whether it is resectable or unresectable.

If the cancer is resectable, you will follow the same neoadjuvant treatment as those who didn't have a dissection (**see Guide 11**, Chapter 6). Then you will have an excision of the recurrent melanoma and systemic adjuvant treatment after that.

Possible treatments include:

- One of the following preferred treatments: nivolumab, pembrolizumab, dabrafenib/trametinib or other BRAF or MEK inhibitors for people with *BRAF* V600 mutation
- Ipilimumab (if you already had anti-PD-1 therapy)
- Clinical trial, in some cases

You might also have one or both of the following:

- Locoregional radiation therapy to nodal basin if you have a higher risk of another recurrence
- Observation as part of follow up care.

For more information on follow-up care, see *Chapter 9: Follow-up care.*

Another option is to omit neoadjuvant therapy and go straight to surgery to remove the recurrent cancer. And if you hadn't received a TLND before, then you can have a TLND at this point. From here on, you will have the same systemic adjuvant therapy mentioned above.

Unresectable disease

Whether or not you had a lymph node removal before, if the cancer is unresectable, then the preferred treatment is the same: systemic therapy (**see Guide 16**, Chapter 8). Additional options include palliative radiation therapy, intralesional T-VEC, and/or best supportive care.

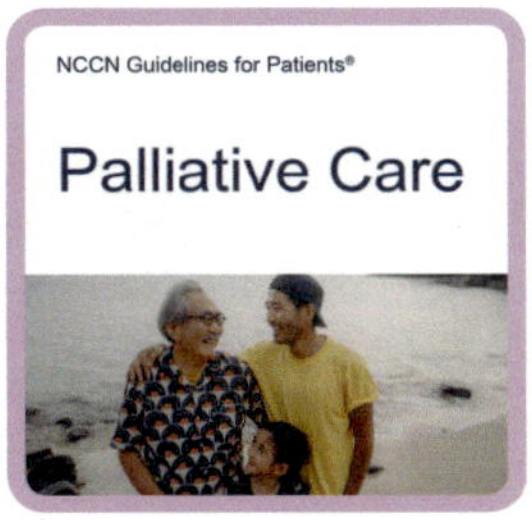

For more information about palliative care, see *NCCN Guidelines for Patients: Palliative Care* at NCCN.org/patientguidelines and on the NCCN Patient Guides for Cancer app.

There are also many clinical trials available for unresectable stage 3 and 4 melanoma. Ask your provider about available clinical trials for the stage of disease you have.

Be your own advocate. Talk to someone who has gone through the same thing as you. Ask a lot of questions, even the ones you are afraid to ask. You have to protect yourself and ensure you make the best decisions for you, and get the best care for your particular situation.”

What's next

In this chapter you learned about the different types of recurrence, which is when melanoma returns. If the recurrent melanoma is considered metastatic, read the next chapter, *Treatment for stage 4: Metastatic disease*. If it's not metastatic, then you will receive follow-up care. Read *Chapter 9: Follow-up care* for more information on your care, genetic risks and testing, and how you can prevent and spot melanoma.

Key points

- When melanoma recurs, it often appears as lumps under the skin or in the lymph nodes.
- True scar recurrence refers to skin tumors that formed from cancer cells that remained near the surgery scar.
- Treatment for true scar recurrence consists of surgery to remove the tumor and possibly lymph nodes. After surgery, you may receive adjuvant therapy.
- Local satellite recurrence and in-transit recurrence both mean the cancer has returned in the lymph vessels.
- Treatment options for local satellite recurrence are based on whether surgery is an option. If there are no signs of cancer after treatment, you may receive more treatment to improve outcomes or start observation.
- Nodal recurrence means melanoma was found in your lymph nodes.
- Treatment for nodal recurrence depends on whether or not the cancer is removable by surgery. If surgery is not an option, the preferred treatment is systemic therapy.

Questions to ask

- Is the cancer considered metastatic?
- Do my lymph nodes need to be removed?
- Am I eligible for a clinical trial?
- What is my risk for another recurrence?
- How do I get a second opinion?

8

Treatment for stage 4: Metastatic disease

Stage 4 cancer, also called metastatic cancer, is melanoma that has spread far from where it started. Metastatic melanoma most often spreads to distant lymph nodes, the brain, bones, liver, lungs, or gastrointestinal (GI) tract.

It is important to know that stage 4 melanoma is treatable. Find a care team that is experienced in treating the type and stage of cancer and also explore clinical trial options. Always ask questions. This will increase your chances of getting the best possible outcome.

Metastatic melanoma may be treated with multiple lines of systemic therapy. The first treatment given is referred to as first-line therapy. Second-line therapy is the second treatment used. If more lines of therapy are needed, other second-line options may be tried. **See Guide 16** for systemic therapy options for metastatic melanoma.

Preferred regimens work better, are safer, or cost less than other options. Your medical oncologist may not prescribe a preferred regimen. Ask why because there are different reasons for this decision.

Non-preferred regimens also have benefits for people with melanoma. They may extend life, delay cancer growth, or reduce symptoms.

Be sure to ask your care team if you have questions about any of your options.

Tests

Tests to evaluate the extent of stage 4 melanoma may involve one or more of the following:

- Core biopsy (preferred) or fine-needle aspiration, incisional (partial) biopsy, or excisional (complete) biopsy
- Lactate dehydrogenase (LDH) testing
- Imaging to see how much the disease has spread and to check cancer signs or symptoms
- *BRAF* mutation testing, if not already done

Guide 15 Possible treatment for metastatic melanoma
Surgery (resection)
Stereotactic ablative therapy
T-VEC/intralesional therapy
Systemic therapy
Palliative resection
Radiation therapy
Supportive care
Observation

Limited metastases

When cancer has spread to only a few distant sites, it is called limited metastatic (or oligometastatic) disease. Your care team will meet with you to discuss primary treatment, which could include options like:

- Surgery (resection)
- Stereotactic radiation therapy, which uses special equipment to position the person and precisely deliver radiation to a tumor
- T-VEC injections into accessible tumors

An additional option is systemic therapy, which is generally recommended either before (neoadjuvant) or after (adjuvant) the removal or treatment of oligometastatic melanoma (**see Guide 16**).

After surgery, radiation, or injections

After treatment for metastatic disease, your team will assess if there are still signs of cancer. If there are no remaining cancer signs, you may be treated with adjuvant therapy or start follow-up care described in Chapter 9. Preferred adjuvant therapy options are:

- Nivolumab
- Pembrolizumab
- Nivolumab/ipilimumab (only IV nivolumab, not injectable, can be combined with ipilimumab)

Other recommended therapy, if you have *BRAF* V600 mutation:

- Dabrafenib/trametinib
- Vemurafenib/cobimetinib
- Encorafenib/binimetinib

In some cases, ipilimumab might be used as adjuvant therapy if you already had anti-PD-1 therapy.

If cancer remains in your body (called residual disease) after any treatment, see the next section on widely disseminated metastases (spread) for treatment options.

After systemic therapy as primary treatment

If you received systemic therapy for oligometastatic melanoma, you will have imaging tests to assess whether the therapy worked.

- If the cancer has spread, see treatment options for widely disseminated metastases.
- If the cancer stayed the same, you may have a resection. If there are no signs of cancer, after surgery, you may receive the same adjuvant therapy mentioned above.
- If there is still disease after surgery, then you will have the treatment for widely disseminated disease.

Widely disseminated metastases

Widely disseminated metastases refers to cancer that has spread to many distant sites. It is unresectable, which means it cannot be completely removed with surgery.

Guide 16
Systemic therapy for metastatic melanoma

Regimens	First-line therapy	Second-line therapy
Nivolumab/ipilimumab*	● (preferred)	● (preferred)
Nivolumab and relatlimab-rmbw	● (preferred)	● (preferred)
Pembrolizumab	● (preferred)	● (preferred)
Nivolumab	● (preferred)	● (preferred)
Dabrafenib/trametinib or vemurafenib/cobimetinib or encorafenib/binimetinib for *BRAF* V600 mutation	● (not preferred)	● (preferred)
Lifileucel (tumor-infiltrating lymphocyte therapy)		● (preferred)
Pembrolizumab/low-dose ipilimumab	● (not preferred)	● (preferred)
Ipilimumab		● (not preferred)
High-dose IL-2		● (not preferred)
Imatinib, dasatinib, nilotinib, or ripretinib for *KIT* mutations		● (not preferred)
Crizotinib or entrectinib for *ROS1* fusions		● (not preferred)
Larotrectinib or entrectinib for *NTRK* fusions		● (not preferred)
Trametinib for *BRAF* fusions		● (not preferred)
Binimetinib for *NRAS* mutation		● (not preferred)
Pembrolizumab/lenvatinib		● (not preferred)
Ipilimumab/intralesional T-VEC		● (not preferred)
Dabrafenib/trametinib plus pembrolizumab or vemurafenib/cobimetinib plus atezolizumab for *BRAF* V600 mutation		● (not preferred)
Chemotherapy		● (not preferred)

● preferred option ● not a preferred option

*only IV nivolumab, not the injectable form, is approved to be used with ipilimumab

Treatment of brain metastases

The first step in treating widely disseminated metastases is to learn if the cancer has reached your brain. Brain metastases are often treated first to prevent serious health problems.

Your care team will meet to discuss treatment options with you. Melanoma experts recommend that the team include a neurosurgeon, radiation oncologist, and medical oncologist. Treatment of brain metastases usually includes both systemic therapy listed in Guide 16 and local treatment to the brain.

For local treatment, surgery is preferred if large brain metastases are causing symptoms or if there is a single metastasis. You may receive radiation therapy after surgery. The preferred radiation method is stereotactic radiosurgery (SRS). This is therapy that uses a high dose of radiation directly into the tumor. If SRS or stereotactic radiation therapy (SRT) are not options, whole brain radiation therapy may be considered.

Sometimes, brain metastases are treated with the goal of relieving symptoms and not removing the cancer. This is called palliative care. Palliative options include:

- Corticosteroids to relieve swelling
- Anticonvulsant therapy to control seizures
- Bevacizumab to help with quality of life

Treatment of body metastases

Treatment options for metastatic melanoma not in the brain include:

- Systemic therapy (preferred)
- Palliative resection and/or radiation therapy
- Intralesional T-VEC injections to treat metastatic skin lesions
- Best supportive/palliative care

For more information about palliative care, see *NCCN Guidelines for Patients: Palliative Care* available at NCCN.org/patientguidelines and on the NCCN Patient Guides for Cancer app.

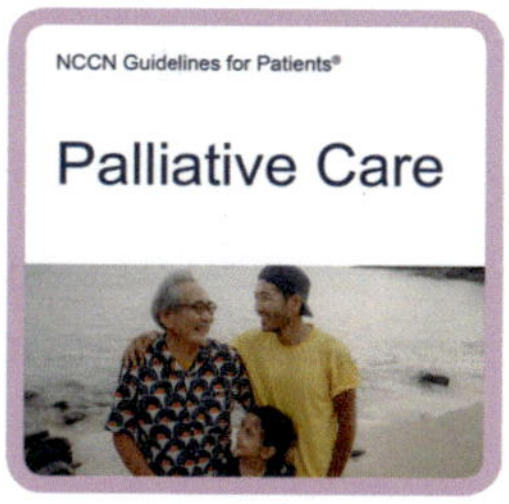

What's next

In this chapter, you learned about stage 4 metastatic melanoma. Cancer that spreads can be treated in a variety of ways. The next chapter about follow-up care includes information on the type of exams you might receive on a regular basis and how to prevent and spot future skin cancers.

Key points

- Stage 4 cancer, also referred to as metastatic cancer, is cancer that has spread from where it started to distant parts of the body.
- Metastatic melanoma is treatable and has many options.
- Cancer that has spread to only a few distant sites is referred to as limited metastatic disease.
- Limited metastatic disease is considered resectable, which means it can be treated by surgery.
- Widely disseminated metastatic disease refers to cancer that has spread to many distant sites.
- Brain metastases are often treated with both systemic therapy and local treatment.
- The preferred treatment for body metastases is systemic therapy.

Questions to ask

- What is your experience treating metastatic melanoma?
- How many of your patients have had complications? What were the complications?
- Who will manage my day-to-day care?
- Is a clinical trial an option for me?
- I would like a second opinion. Is there someone you can recommend?

"There are always options. You know your body best and must advocate for what would best meet your needs. Second and third opinions should always be encouraged and if something doesn't feel right, speak up and take action."

9
Follow-up care

After treatment for melanoma, your care team will want to check you for any new skin cancers – often called follow-up or monitoring. They can also help you take the best care of your skin and help prevent melanoma from coming back. This chapter explains ongoing care for everyone who's had melanoma.

Melanoma tests

Skin and lymph node exams

Your provider may do exams on your skin and lymph nodes **at least** once a year depending on the melanoma stage. Your doctor should also explain how you can do self-exams of your skin and lymph nodes at home. It's important to regularly look for any new, changing, or unusual spots on both sun-exposed and non-exposed skin.

What you can do:

- **Examine your skin regularly** — If you spot anything that looks out of the ordinary or doesn't look normal, get it checked out as soon as possible.
- **See your health care provider annually for a skin exam** — Ask for a full-body skin exam by a provider, like a dermatologist, at least once a year. You may want to consider a skin exam more often if you are at higher risk for skin cancer.

Skin devices

Your care team might use medical tools to check for skin cancer, such as:

- **Dermatoscope** — a hand-held device to provide a closer look at suspicious lesions
- **Total-body photography** — to help with ongoing monitoring of moles on the skin

These tools are especially important if you develop atypical-looking moles (moles that are called dysplastic under a microscope) or other suspicious skin surfaces. Though atypical moles are usually non-cancerous, they can put you at greater risk of developing future melanoma.

Imaging tests

If you had a past lymph node exam that showed cancer, your doctor might consider more imaging scans (for example, an ultrasound or CT scan). This could be followed by a more thorough imaging or biopsy if your provider feels it is needed.

How often you receive follow-up testing depends on how likely it is that the cancer will return, which can also depend on your family history of melanoma, if you have a high mole count, or if you have any atypical-looking moles.

Genes and genetic risk

Genes are the instructions in cells for making new cells and controlling how cells behave. An abnormal change in these instructions, called a gene mutation, may cause cells to grow and multiply out of control. Gene mutations can lead to genetic conditions like cancer.

Melanoma is a type of cancer that can run in families. About 1 in 10 people with melanoma have a family member who has or has had melanoma. Some families get melanoma because they share the same skin type or history of sun exposure. Other families share genes that put them at risk for melanoma.

Inherited genes that increase melanoma risk may also increase the risk of other cancers. You may have hereditary melanoma if you have a family history of:

- Skin (cutaneous) melanoma or eye (uveal) melanoma, especially among multiple blood relatives
- Pancreatic, kidney, bladder, gastrointestinal, or breast cancer
- Astrocytoma (cancer of the brain or spinal cord)
- Mesothelioma (cancer of the tissue that covers the lungs and other internal organs)

There are several abnormal (mutated) genes related to hereditary melanoma. They include:

- *CDKN2A* mutation for melanoma, which is the most common gene mutation for melanoma. It is also called p16INK4A or MTS1. It often means that many cases of melanoma that were found at an early age run in your family.
- The melanocortin-1 receptor (*MC1R*) gene, which helps determine your skin's color. MC1R can determine if you or your family members have red hair and/or light skin, which increases your risk for developing melanoma.
- *BAP1* gene mutations, which can cause uveal and, less often, cutaneous melanoma.

Genetic testing

Your clinical and family history might call for multigene testing, which can help your care team know if you have a higher genetic risk for developing melanoma and other cancers. This information can help guide recommendations for early detection and monitoring in both you and your family members.

You might be referred for genetic counseling and p16/CDKN2A testing if you or someone in your family has a history of 2 or more instances of diagnoses of invasive cutaneous melanoma. You might also be referred if you or someone in your family has a history of 2 or more non-skin cancers especially uveal melanoma, pancreatic, kidney, bladder, gastrointestinal and/or breast cancer, mesothelioma, and/or astrocytoma.

Multigene panel testing that includes CDKN2A may also be recommended if you have a relative diagnosed with pancreatic cancer. Testing for other genes that can harbor melanoma-predisposing mutations may also be needed.

For more information about genetic testing, *see NCCN Guidelines for Patients: Genetic Testing for Hereditary Breast, Ovarian, Pancreatic, and Prostate Cancers* available at NCCN.org/patientguidelines and on the NCCN Patient Guides for Cancer app.

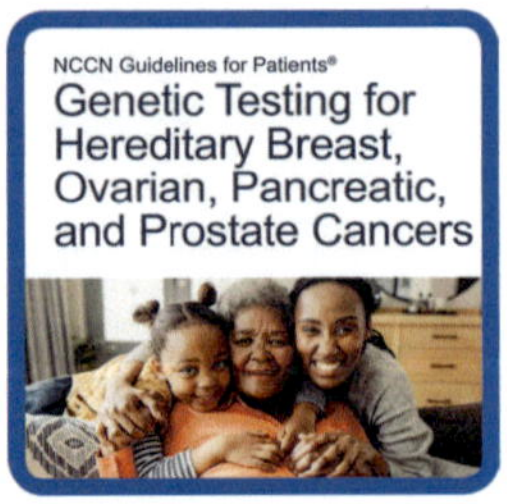

Early detection: ABCDE rule

In between your regular visits with your provider, following the ABCDE rule is a good way to help detect the signs of melanoma. Check moles or spots on your own in front of a mirror (a handheld mirror can help, too) or with a partner and keep this rule in mind:

- **Asymmetry** – This means the mole or spot is not uniform and one half doesn't match the other half.
- **Border** – The edges of a spot seem irregular and are difficult to define.
- **Color** – The color of the spot is not the same throughout (may be brown, black, or sometimes with patches of pink, red, white, or blue).
- **Diameter** – The spot is larger than 6 mm across (about the size of a pencil eraser).
- **Evolving** – The spot or mole changes its size, shape, or color over time.

Early detection of melanoma: ABCDE rule

For skin self-exams, always follow the ABCDE rule to detect unusual moles.

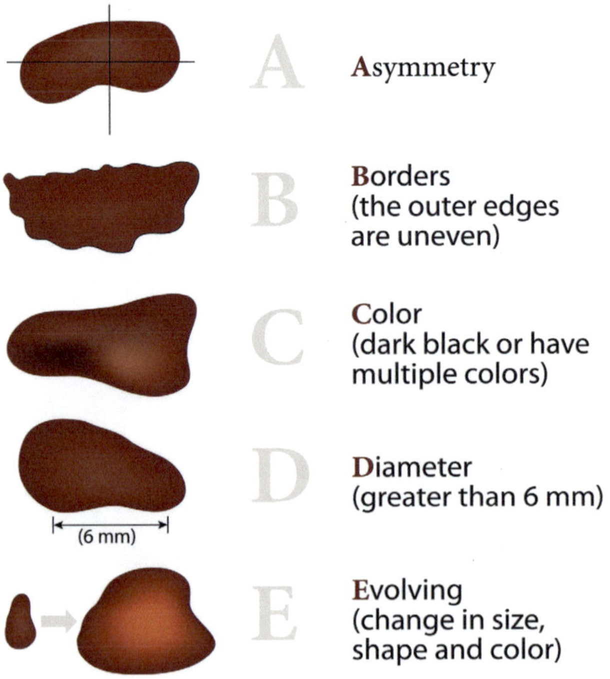

Preventing melanoma

You can take steps to help stop melanoma cells from reforming. Taking preventive action is important if you are at higher risk, have sun sensitivity, or a lighter complexion:

- **Reduce UV (ultraviolet) radiation exposure –** This means reducing your exposure to the sun and avoiding the use of indoor tanning beds and other devices.
- **Prevent sun damage –** Limit your sun exposure between peak hours of 10:00 am and 4:00 pm.
- **Wear protective clothing –** This includes a wide-brim hat, clothes made with UV-protective fabric, and sunglasses.
- **Use sunscreen –** Choose a broad-spectrum sunscreen with a sun protection factor (SPF) of at least 30. Reapply it at least once every 2 hours. Sunscreen should be applied 15 minutes before going outside to be most effective.
- **Check your skin regularly –** This includes both self-examinations and skin exams by a health care provider.

Limit time in the sun

Use caution when spending time outdoors. Reduce your risk of skin cancer by limiting sun exposure, wearing protective clothing, and using sunscreen.

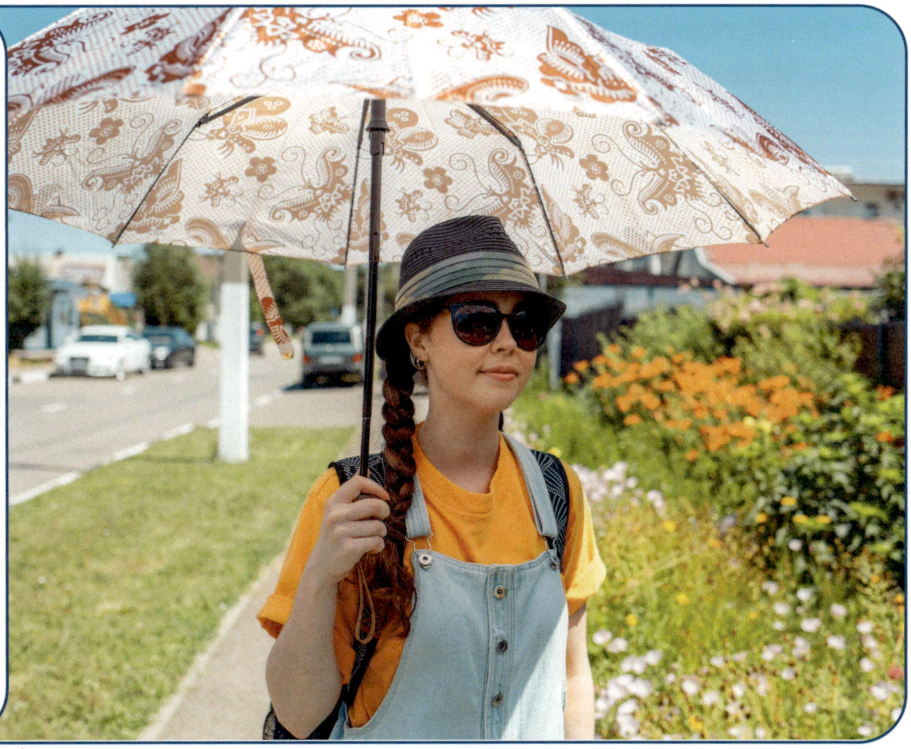

Key points

- Your provider may expect to examine your skin and lymph nodes at least once a year.
- How often you receive follow-up testing depends on how likely it is that the cancer will return.
- Your provider should also explain how you can do self-exams of your skin and your lymph nodes.
- Your care team might use devices to help detect new melanomas early.
- If you had a past lymph node exam that showed cancer, your doctor might consider more imaging.
- You might be referred for genetic counseling if genetic tests show 2 or more instances of cancer diagnoses in your family.
- You can take several steps to help stop melanoma cells from reforming, especially if you have sun sensitivity or lighter skin.

“I was lucky. I had melanoma twice: once on my leg and once on my back. If it weren't for my doctor doing the skin exam, I would not have known about the one on my back.”

Questions to ask

- If I find an unusual spot, what should I do?
- Do I need genetic testing?
- What SPF is best for me?
- Can you recommend trusted brands of sunscreen?
- Do you have any recommendations for local melanoma support groups?

10
Other resources

Want to learn more? Here's how you can get additional help.

What else to know

This book can help you improve your cancer care. It plainly explains expert recommendations and suggests questions to ask your care team. But it's not the only resource that you have.

You're welcome to receive as much information and help as you need. Many people are interested in learning more about:

- The details of melanoma and treatment
- Being a part of a care team
- Getting financial help
- Finding a care provider who is an expert in their field
- Coping with health problems

What else to do

Your health care center can help you with next steps. They often have on-site resources to help meet your needs and find answers to your questions. Health care centers can also inform you of resources in your community.

In addition to help from your providers, the resources listed in the next section provide support for many people like yourself. Look through the list and visit the provided websites to learn more about these organizations.

Where to get help

AIM at Melanoma
AIMatMelanoma.org

AIM at Skin Cancer
AIMatSkinCancer.org

Cancer*Care*
Cancercare.org

Cancer Hope Network
cancerhopenetwork.org

Clear Cell Sarcoma
Clearcellsarcoma.org

Imerman Angels
Imermanangels.org

Melanoma Research Alliance
Curemelanoma.org

Melanoma Research Foundation
melanoma.org

My Faulty Gene
Myfaultygene.org

National Coalition for Cancer Survivorship
canceradvocacy.org

Save Your Skin Foundation
saveyourskin.ca

The Skin Cancer Foundation
skincancer.org

Triage Cancer
Triagecancer.org

Questions to ask

- Who can I talk to about help with housing, food, and other basic needs?
- What assistance is available for transportation, childcare, and home care?
- How much will I have to pay for treatment?
- What help is available to pay for medicines and other treatment?
- What other services are available to me and my caregivers?

We want your feedback!

Our goal is to provide helpful and easy-to-understand information on cancer. Take our survey to let us know what we got right and what we could do better.
NCCN.org/patients/feedback

Words to know

ABCDE rule
A memory device to recognize the characteristics of moles or skin lesions that might be cancer.

adjuvant treatment
Treatment (usually medicine or radiation) that is given after the main (primary) treatment.

advanced melanoma
Cancer that has spread beyond the area near the main tumor.

anesthesia
A drug or other substance that causes a controlled loss of feeling or awareness with or without loss of wakefulness.

asymmetry
A characteristic of possible skin cancer in which one half or side of a mole does not match the other half or side.

best supportive care
Health care for the symptoms of cancer and the side effects of cancer treatment. Also sometimes called palliative care.

biopsy
Removal of small amounts of tissue from your body to test for disease.

***BRAF* mutations**
BRAF mutations can cause normal cells to become cancerous. They are most commonly found in melanomas but can occur in other forms of cancer.

Breslow thickness
A measure of how deep the melanoma tumor has grown into the skin.

broad-spectrum sunscreen
A substance that protects the skin from the sun by blocking 2 types of harmful ultraviolet (UV) rays — UVA and UVB.

cancer stage
Rating or description of the growth and spread of cancer in the body.

chemotherapy
Drugs that kill fast-growing cells, including normal cells and cancer cells.

clinical stage
A rating of the extent of melanoma in the body based on the physical exam and biopsy of the first (primary) tumor.

clinical trial
Research on a test or treatment to assess its safety or how well it works.

complete lymph node dissection (CLND)
A type of surgery that removes the remaining lymph nodes after a positive sentinel lymph node biopsy. Also called completion lymph node dissection.

computed tomography (CT) scan
A test that uses x-rays from many angles to make a picture of the inside of the body.

contrast
A dye put into your body to make clearer pictures during tests that take pictures of the inside of the body.

dermal mitotic rate
A measure of how many cancer cells are growing and dividing in the dermis.

dermatologist
A doctor who's an expert in skin diseases.

dermis
The second layer of skin that is beneath the top layer (epidermis).

distant metastasis
The spread of cancer cells to a part of the body far away from the first (primary) melanoma tumor.

DNA (deoxyribonucleic acid)
A long molecule that contains our unique genetic code.

epidermis
The outer layer of skin.

excision
Removal by surgery.

excisional biopsy
Surgery that removes the entire skin tumor or abnormal-looking area (lesion) to test for cancer cells.

fine-needle aspiration biopsy
Use of a thin needle to remove fluid or tissue from the body to be tested for disease.

follow-up tests
Tests done after treatment to check for signs of cancer return (recurrence) or spread (metastasis).

general anesthesia
A drug-induced, sleep-like state for pain relief.

genes
A set of coded instructions in cells for making new cells and controlling how cells behave.

imaging
Any radiology test that makes pictures (images) of the insides of the body.

immunotherapy
Treatment that uses the immune system to kill cancer cells.

infusion
A method of putting fluids, including drugs, into the bloodstream.

in-transit metastases
The spread of skin cancer through a lymph vessel.

lymphedema
Swelling due to buildup of lymph fluid in the fatty tissue just under the skin near the surgery site.

lymph node
A small bean-shaped structure that is part of the body's immune system.

lymph node basin
A group of lymph nodes that receives and filters lymph that flows from a certain area of the body.

lymph vessels
Similar to blood vessels, lymph vessels are thin-walled and tube-like but carry a fluid called lymph.

metastasis
The spread of cancer cells from the first (primary) tumor to a new site.

microsatellites
Tiny tumor deposits that have spread to lymph vessels in the skin near the first melanoma tumor and can only be seen with a microscope.

neoadjuvant treatment
Treatment (usually medicine) that is given before the main (primary) treatment, usually surgery.

palliative care
Specialized medical care aimed at increasing quality of life and reducing pain and discomfort for people with serious, complex illness.

radiation therapy
A treatment that uses high-energy rays to kill cancer cells.

recurrence
The return of cancer after a cancer-free period.

resectable
Cancer able to be removed (resected) by surgery.

sentinel lymph node biopsy (SLNB)
Surgery to find and remove a sentinel lymph node to see if it contains cancer cells.

stereotactic radiosurgery (SRS)
A treatment that gives a single large dose of radiation concentrated on a tumor, while limiting the dose to surrounding organs.

sun protection factor (SPF)
A number that indicates how well the sunscreen filters out UV rays and protects skin against sunburn.

talimogene laherparepvec (T-VEC)
Treatment that uses a virus to infect and kill cancer cells while avoiding normal, healthy cells.

targeted therapy
A drug treatment that identifies and attacks a specific feature of cancer cells with less harm to normal cells.

tumor-infiltrating lymphocyte (TIL) therapy
Treatment where tumor-infiltrating lymphocytes are removed from the person's tumor, grown in a laboratory, and given back to the person by infusion.

ulceration
A break in the skin like an open sore.

unresectable
Cancer that is not able to be surgically removed.

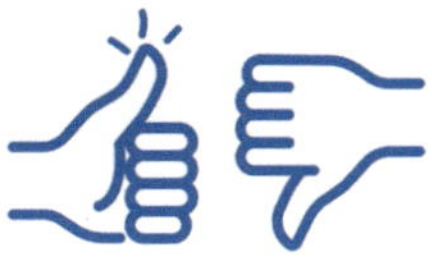

Let us know what you think!

Please take a moment to complete an online survey about the NCCN Guidelines for Patients.
NCCN.org/patients/response

NCCN Contributors

This patient guide is based on the NCCN Clinical Practice Guidelines in Oncology (NCCN Guidelines®) for Melanoma: Cutaneous, Version 2.2025. It was adapted, reviewed, and published with help from the following people:

Dorothy A. Shead, MS
Senior Director
Patient Information Operations

Christine McLaughlin
Medical Writer

Susan Kidney
Senior Graphic Design Specialist

The NCCN Clinical Practice Guidelines in Oncology (NCCN Guidelines®) for Melanoma: Cutaneous, Version 2.2025 were developed by the following NCCN Panel Members:

*Susan M. Swetter, MD/Chair
Stanford Cancer Institute

*Douglas Johnson, MD, MSCI
Vice-Chair
Vanderbilt-Ingram Cancer Center

Mark R. Albertini, MD
University of Wisconsin
Carbone Cancer Center

Christopher A. Barker, MD
Memorial Sloan Kettering Cancer Center

*Sarah Bateni, MD, MAS
O'Neal Comprehensive
Cancer Center at UAB

Joel Baumgartner, MD
UC San Diego Moores Cancer Center

Shailender Bhatia, MD
Fred Hutchinson Cancer Center

Christopher Bichakjian, MD
University of Michigan Rogel Cancer Center

Genevieve Boland, MD, PhD
Mass General Cancer Center

Sunandana Chandra, MD, MS
Robert H. Lurie Comprehensive Cancer
Center of Northwestern University

Bartosz Chmielowski, MD, PhD
UCLA Jonsson
Comprehensive Cancer Center

Dominick DiMaio, MD
Fred & Pamela Buffett Cancer Center

Roxana Dronca, MD
Mayo Clinic Comprehensive Cancer Center

Ryan C. Fields, MD
Siteman Cancer Center at Barnes-
Jewish Hospital and Washington
University School of Medicine

Martin D. Fleming, MD
The University of Tennessee
Health Science Center

*Anjela Galan, MD
Yale Cancer Center/Smilow Cancer Hospital

*Samantha Guild
AIM at Melanoma

Siwen Hu-Lieskovan, MD, PhD
Huntsman Cancer Institute
at the University of Utah

John Hyngstrom, MD
Huntsman Cancer Institute
at the University of Utah

Giorgos Karakousis, MD
Abramson Cancer Center
at the University of Pennsylvania

Kari Kendra, MD, PhD
The Ohio State University Comprehensive
Cancer Center - James Cancer Hospital
and Solove Research Institute

Maija Kiuru, MD, PhD
UC Davis Comprehensive Cancer Center

Julie R. Lange, MD, ScM
Johns Hopkins Kimmel Cancer Center

Ryan Lanning, MD, PhD
University of Colorado Cancer Center

Theodore Logan, MD
Indiana University Melvin and Bren Simon
Comprehensive Cancer Center

Daniel Olson, MD
The UChicago Medicine
Comprehensive Cancer Center

Anthony J. Olszanski, MD, RPh
Fox Chase Cancer Center

Patrick A. Ott, MD, PhD
Dana-Farber/Brigham and
Women's Cancer Center

Igor Puzanov, MD, MSCI
Roswell Park Comprehensive Cancer Center

Luke Rothermel, MD, MPH
Case Comprehensive Cancer Center/
University Hospitals Seidman Cancer Center
and Cleveland Clinic Taussig Cancer Institute

April K. Salama, MD
Duke Cancer Institute

Rohit Sharma, MD
UT Southwestern Simmons
Comprehensive Cancer Center

Joseph Skitzki, MD
Roswell Park Comprehensive Cancer Center

Katy Tsai, MD
UCSF Helen Diller Family
Comprehensive Cancer Center

Evan Wuthrick, MD
Moffitt Cancer Center

Yan Xing, MD, PhD
City of Hope National Medical Center

NCCN

Sara Espinosa, PhD
Oncology Scientist/Medical Writer

Nicole McMillian, MS
Senior Guidelines Coordinator

* Reviewed this patient guide. For disclosures, visit NCCN.org/disclosures.

NCCN Cancer Centers

Abramson Cancer Center
at the University of Pennsylvania
Philadelphia, Pennsylvania
800.789.7366 • pennmedicine.org/cancer

Case Comprehensive Cancer Center/
University Hospitals Seidman Cancer Center and
Cleveland Clinic Taussig Cancer Institute
Cleveland, Ohio
UH Seidman Cancer Center
800.641.2422 • uhhospitals.org/services/cancer-services
CC Taussig Cancer Institute
866.223.8100 • my.clevelandclinic.org/departments/cancer
Case CCC
216.844.8797 • case.edu/cancer

City of Hope National Medical Center
Duarte, California
800.826.4673 • cityofhope.org

Dana-Farber/Brigham and Women's Cancer Center |
Mass General Cancer Center
Boston, Massachusetts
877.442.3324 • youhaveus.org
617.726.5130 • massgeneral.org/cancer-center

Duke Cancer Institute
Durham, North Carolina
888.275.3853 • dukecancerinstitute.org

Fox Chase Cancer Center
Philadelphia, Pennsylvania
888.369.2427 • foxchase.org

Fred & Pamela Buffett Cancer Center
Omaha, Nebraska
402.559.5600 • unmc.edu/cancercenter

Fred Hutchinson Cancer Center
Seattle, Washington
206.667.5000 • fredhutch.org

Huntsman Cancer Institute at the University of Utah
Salt Lake City, Utah
800.824.2073 • healthcare.utah.edu/huntsmancancerinstitute

Indiana University Melvin and Bren Simon
Comprehensive Cancer Center
Indianapolis, Indiana
888.600.4822 • www.cancer.iu.edu

Johns Hopkins Kimmel Cancer Center
Baltimore, Maryland
410.955.8964
www.hopkinskimmelcancercenter.org

Mayo Clinic Comprehensive Cancer Center
Phoenix/Scottsdale, Arizona
Jacksonville, Florida
Rochester, Minnesota
480.301.8000 • Arizona
904.953.0853 • Florida
507.538.3270 • Minnesota
mayoclinic.org/cancercenter

Memorial Sloan Kettering Cancer Center
New York, New York
800.525.2225 • mskcc.org

Moffitt Cancer Center
Tampa, Florida
888.663.3488 • moffitt.org

O'Neal Comprehensive Cancer Center at UAB
Birmingham, Alabama
800.822.0933 • uab.edu/onealcancercenter

Robert H. Lurie Comprehensive Cancer Center
of Northwestern University
Chicago, Illinois
866.587.4322 • cancer.northwestern.edu

Roswell Park Comprehensive Cancer Center
Buffalo, New York
877.275.7724 • roswellpark.org

Siteman Cancer Center at Barnes-Jewish Hospital
and Washington University School of Medicine
St. Louis, Missouri
800.600.3606 • siteman.wustl.edu

St. Jude Children's Research Hospital/
The University of Tennessee Health Science Center
Memphis, Tennessee
866.278.5833 • stjude.org
901.448.5500 • uthsc.edu

Stanford Cancer Institute
Stanford, California
877.668.7535 • cancer.stanford.edu

The Ohio State University Comprehensive Cancer Center -
James Cancer Hospital and Solove Research Institute
Columbus, Ohio
800.293.5066 • cancer.osu.edu

The UChicago Medicine Comprehensive Cancer Center
Chicago, Illinois
773.702.1000 • uchicagomedicine.org/cancer

The University of Texas MD Anderson Cancer Center
Houston, Texas
844.269.5922 • mdanderson.org

UC Davis Comprehensive Cancer Center
Sacramento, California
916.734.5959 • 800.770.9261
health.ucdavis.edu/cancer

UC San Diego Moores Cancer Center
La Jolla, California
858.822.6100 • cancer.ucsd.edu

UCLA Jonsson Comprehensive Cancer Center
Los Angeles, California
310.825.5268 • uclahealth.org/cancer

UCSF Helen Diller Family
Comprehensive Cancer Center
San Francisco, California
800.689.8273 • cancer.ucsf.edu

University of Colorado Cancer Center
Aurora, Colorado
720.848.0300 • coloradocancercenter.org

University of Michigan Rogel Cancer Center
Ann Arbor, Michigan
800.865.1125 • rogelcancercenter.org

University of Wisconsin Carbone Cancer Center
Madison, Wisconsin
608.265.1700 • uwhealth.org/cancer

UT Southwestern Simmons
Comprehensive Cancer Center
Dallas, Texas
214.648.3111 • utsouthwestern.edu/simmons

Vanderbilt-Ingram Cancer Center
Nashville, Tennessee
877.936.8422 • vicc.org

Yale Cancer Center/Smilow Cancer Hospital
New Haven, Connecticut
855.4.SMILOW • yalecancercenter.org

share with us.

Take our survey and help make the NCCN Guidelines for Patients better for everyone!

NCCN.org/patients/comments

Notes

Index

Made in the USA
Monee, IL
05 November 2026

67382285R00057